H. Sattler U. Harland

Arthro-sonography

Foreword by Hans Rettig

With 144 Figures in 271 Parts
and 6 Tables

Springer-Verlag Berlin Heidelberg New York
London Paris Tokyo Hong Kong

Dr. HORST SATTLER
Wicker-Klinik, Kaiser-Friedrich-Promenade 47
6380 Bad Homburg
Federal Republic of Germany

Dr. ULRICH HARLAND
Orthopädische Klinik
Paul-Meimberg-Straße 3, 6300 Gießen
Federal Republic of Germany

Translated by TERRY C. TELGER

Translation of "Arthrosonographie", 1988
ISBN-13: 978-3-642-73869-2 Verlag Berlin Heidelberg New York

Library of Congress Cataloging in Publication Data
Sattler, H. (Horst), 1947–   [Arthrosonographie. English]
Arthrosonography / H. Sattler, U. Harland ; foreword by Hans Rettig ; [translated by Terry C. Telger].
p.   cm. Translation of: Arthrosonographie.
Includes bibliographical references.
ISBN-13: 978-3-642-73869-2   e-ISBN-13: 978-3-642-73867-8
DOI: 10.1007/ 978-3-642-73867-8
1. Joints - Ultrasonic imaging. 2. Joints - Diseases - Diagnosis.
I. Harland, U. (Ulrich) II. Title.
RC932.S2713   1990   616.7'207543 - dc20   89-21773

© Springer-Verlag Berlin Heidelberg 1990
Softcover reprint of the hardcover 1st edition 1990

Typesetting : Appl, Wemding
2121/3145-543210   Printed on acid-free paper

*Amid all the enthusiasm
for modern medical technology,
we must not forget
the needs and sufferings
of our patients.*

*This book is dedicated to the patients who,
through their patience and cooperation,
contributed to the advance
of this diagnostic method.*

Foreword

Sonography is a noninvasive diagnostic method that has gained an established place in many branches of medicine.

Although the inability of ultrasound to penetrate bone delayed its application in the orthopedic field, the successful work of R. Graf in the early detection of pediatric hip disorders with ultrasound has served as an impetus for the increasing use of sonography to detect and evaluate abnormalities of the musculoskeletal system.

It is certain that further advances in this modality will be forthcoming, and that sonography will be applied to new lines of investigation in orthopedic diagnosis.

In *Arthrosonography* the authors use concise text and copious illustrations to demonstrate the potential applications of articular ultrasound, its diagnostic capabilities, and technical aspects of the ultrasound examination. Potential pitfalls are also explained.

This book is the logical outcome of the application of diagnostic ultrasound in orthopedics and rheumatology. It covers all basic practical aspects of arthrosonography and will be a valued resource for those concerned with the evaluation of the musculoskeletal system.

HANS RETTIG

Contents

Introduction

The Piezoelectric Effect – The Basis of Modern Sonography

The piezoelectric effect, discovered by the Curie brothers in 1880, is the foundation of modern diagnostic ultrasound. When an electrical voltage is applied to a small, thin crystal plate having an asymmetrical crystal lattice, the plate will respond by undergoing a change in thickness. Accordingly, an alternating voltage will excite the crystal to undergo rhythmic volume changes, which are transmitted to the environment as pressure waves. This effect is reversible, i. e., mechanical deformation of the polar crystal element, caused for example by incident sound waves, will alter the electrical charge on the crystal surface. Because of these phenomena a single crystal element can serve as both a transmitter and a receiver of ultrasound waves, in effect becoming an electromagnetic transducer.

Ultrasound Techniques

A scan: Amplitude-modulated scan: the simplest, one-dimensional sonographic technique.

B scan: Brightness-modulated scan: multiple ultrasound beams are arranged sequentially in one plane to create a two-dimensional image.

TM scan: Time-motion or M-mode display: the echoes produced by a one-dimensional ultrasound beam are recorded continuously over time.

Doppler scan: Exploits the fact that reflected portions of an ultrasound beam undergo a frequency change, or Doppler shift, when they strike a moving interface (such as a pulsating vessel wall).

Compound scan: Older B-scan technique. Can image whole body cross-sections, but the slow scanning process is very sensitive to motion artifacts.

Fast B scan: Known also as real-time scanning, this technique provides rapid image generation in a fraction of a second by a mechanically or electronically controlled scanning process. Organ movements can be directly observed and can help to guide the examination.

Today B-scan techniques are available with:
- mechanical sector scanners;
- electronic sector scanners, called phased arrays;
- mechanical parallel scanners with water coupling;
- electronic parallel scanners, called linear arrays.

General Principles of Diagnostic Ultrasound

Ultrasound waves travel through body tissues in accordance with the acoustic properties of the various biologic media. They behave similarly to light waves in that they can be reflected, scattered, refracted, diffracted, and absorbed.

The longitudinal waves consist of a rhythmic sequence of compressive and tensile stresses. The particles in the medium respond to these stresses by undergoing rhythmic density changes in the direction of the sound propagation. The velocity at which longitudinal sound waves travel through human tissue depends on the type of tissue that is traversed, as shown in Table 1.

The basis for diagnostic ultrasound is the "acoustic interface," or the boundary that exists between two media having different velocities of sound conduction. The acoustic "impedance jump" at the interface has measurable effects on an impinging ultrasound beam. Because acoustic and anatomic interfaces generally coincide, the change in the sound waves at acoustic interfaces can be used to reconstruct an anatomic image. A beam encountering an interface between tissues with very different acoustic impedances will be almost totally reflected. This occurs, for example, at the boundary between connective tissue and aerated lung or between soft-tissue structures and bone. The latter interface is of major importance in arthrosonography. If the acoustic impedances of two contiguous media are known, the reflected and transmitted intensities can be determined. The impedance jump is maximal when the acoustic interface is perpendicular to the incident sound waves.

Table 1. Velocity of sound conduction in different media

Medium	Temperature °C	Frequency MHz	Sound velocity m/s
Water	25	–	1497
Water	25	15	1495
Human tissue	37	2.5	1490–1610
Human tissues			
Mean value	37	2.5	1540
Muscle	24	1.8	1568
Liver	24	1.8	1570
Fat	24	1.8	1476
Brain	24	2.0	1521
Cranial bone	–	0.8	3360

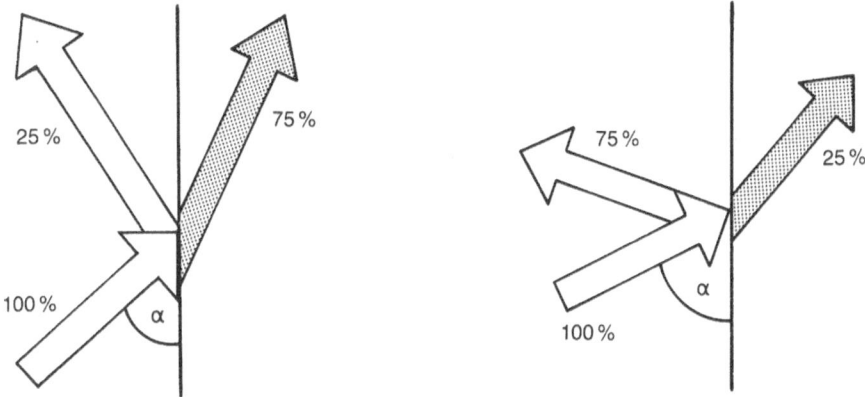

Fig. 1. Effect of reflection and diffraction angles on image production with ultrasound

An impedance difference of only 1% is sufficient to produce a detectable echo that can be used to construct a sonographic image of the tissue interface. Tissues with equal echo densities are "acoustically homogeneous" and are indistinguishable from one another on sonograms.

The following properties of sound waves are of fundamental importance:

1. Reflection
This depends on the difference in the acoustic properties of two adjacent media.

2. Refraction
Ultrasound waves are refracted as they pass from one medium to another medium having a different acoustic density. The degree of refraction can be calculated from the ratio of the sound conduction velocities of the media (Fig. 1).

3. Diffraction
Ultrasound waves travel in a linear path in a homogeneous medium. If an obstacle is placed in the path of the waves, the waves will "bend" around the edge of the obstacle into its acoustic shadow. This phenomenon, called diffraction, is dependent on wavelength and frequency: diffraction decreases as the frequency of the waves is increased.

4. Scatter
Ultrasound waves are scattered when they encounter an interface that is not perpendicular to their direction of incidence. Because virtually all surfaces in biologic media are acoustically "rough," scattering is an important phenomenon in sonography. The degree of scatter is frequency dependent, i.e., the intensity of the scattered sound waves increases with frequency (Fig. 2).

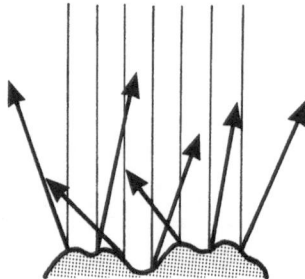

Fig. 2. The scattering of sound waves at irregular interfaces. Since all tissue layers and organ surfaces are acoustically rough, scattered echoes occur in all body regions

5. Absorption

Part of the energy in the ultrasound beam is lost by conversion to heat. It is necessary, therefore, to amplify echoes from deeper tissue layers by a process known as depth gain compensation or time gain compensation in order to correct for the energy lost to absorption.

The penetrating capacity of the ultrasound beam is determined by its resolution, scatter, and absorption and declines with increasing frequency. The progressive weakening of sound intensity by a medium, called attenuation, is measured in decibel units/cm^2 (Table 2).

Fluids do not contain reflective interfaces and therefore appear echo-free, although scattered echoes may be returned by exfoliated cells. Parenchymatous organs, on the other hand, contain abundant echogenic interfaces. The ability to differentiate between echogenic and echo-free areas is one of the distinctive qualities of diagnostic ultrasound.

Because sound waves are not reflected by fluids and thus lose no energy when traversing a fluid medium, "acoustic enhancement" is observed behind purely fluid-filled areas. This phenomenon is characteristic of cysts and effusions.

Time gain compensation. Echoes coming from deeper structures must be modified such that their amplitude will be equivalent to that of more superficial echoes. This can be accomplished either by amplifying the deeper echoes or by weakening the superficial ones. Accordingly, different adjustments of the time gain compensation (TGC) have a major impact on the appearance of anatomic

Table 2. Attenuation of sound intensity in various tissues (1 MHz)

Fat	0.35–0.7
Muscle	1.5–3.0
Liver	0.95
Kidney	1.1
Bone	12.0

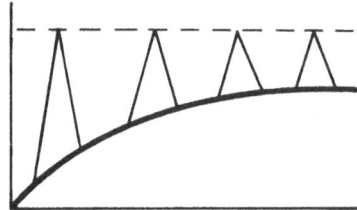

Fig. 3. Time gain compensation: Echoes from deeper structures are amplified to correct for attenuation and achieve a uniform amplitude level for all echoes

structures. The quality of the sonographic image depends critically on an appropriate TGC setting (Fig. 3).

Lateral resolution. The lateral resolution of an ultrasound system depends on the geometry of the transducer, the ultrasound frequency, and the pulse length. It is inversely proportional to the width of the ultrasound beam. In practical terms, lateral resolution denotes the minimum transverse distance between two objects (relative to the direction of the ultrasound beam) at which they can still be recognized as being separate from each other.

Axial resolution. This refers to the minimum longitudinal distance between two objects (relative to the ultrasound beam) that can still be resolved as separate objects. It is limited by the pulse length and increases with the sound frequency.

The ultrasound beam is regarded as consisting of two regions: the near field and the far field. An object is defined most clearly when it lies within the focus, which is at the end of the near field on the axis of the beam (Fig. 4).

Acoustic shadows. When sound waves are reflected and absorbed at an acoustic interface, shadowlike areas may appear behind the interface. Bone, calculi, and calcifications are the most frequent sources of dense acoustic shadows. Much lighter shadows may be cast by gas collections.

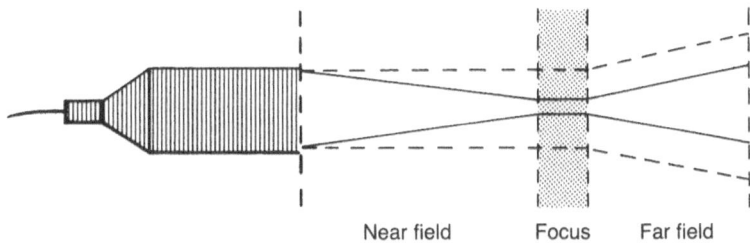

Near field   Focus   Far field

Fig. 4. Schematic representation of the focusing of a sound beam by an acoustic lens

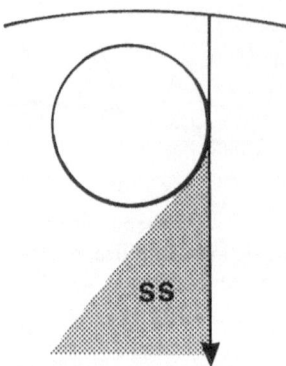

Fig. 5. Diffraction shadow at the edge of a cyst ("magnifying glass" pheonomenon). A diffraction shadow appears when sound waves are diffracted toward the medium with the higher velocity of sound transmission

Acoustic shadows also occur at the edges of cyst walls. This "magnifying glass" phenomenon results from diffraction of the sound beam toward the more conductive material within the cyst (Fig. 5).

Landmarks for Arthrosonography

A coupling medium is applied between the ultrasound transducer and body surface to avoid the total reflection that would otherwise occur at the thin air layer between the transducer and skin.

Every ultrasound examination of the joints should be performed systematically with an effort made to define specific structures in standard, reproducible views. Bony surfaces and large blood vessels provide essential *landmarks* for this process:

1. *Bony contour:* appears as a line or arc of high-level echoes with distal acoustic shadowing.
2. *Blood vessels:* appear as echo-free tubular structures.
3. *Muscle groups:* appear hypoechoic, with muscular septa presenting a feathery or ordered echo pattern.
4. *Hyaline cartilage:* appears as a hypoechoic to echo-free layer directly overlying a highly echogenic bone surface.

Artifacts

Knowledge of potential artifacts is necessary for the correct interpretation of scans. Artifacts are phenomena inherent in the ultrasound system; they cannot be eliminated by instrument adjustments. Artifacts are most commonly seen below bony surfaces.

Reverberations

Ultrasound waves that become "trapped" between two or more parallel interfaces are reflected repeatedly between the interfaces, giving rise to an increasingly attenuated train of echo pulses. The instrument cannot recognize this "beam trapping" phenomenon as such, but portrays the reflective interfaces as a series of parallel lines that become increasingly faint with distance from the transducer. The more parallel interfaces there are, and the more reverberations are set up between them, the greater the number of parallel echoes that appear on the image (Fig.6a).

Hyperbolic Artifacts

Sound waves encountering a highly echogenic interface not only produce a bright central echo but, through "side lobe effects," also give rise to a curved line of smaller echoes very close to the echogenic surface (Fig.6b). These artifacts are most conspicuous in echo-free media.

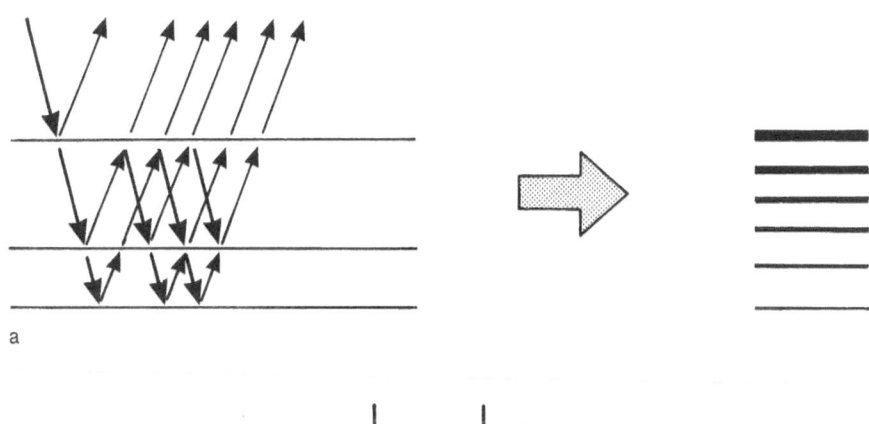

a

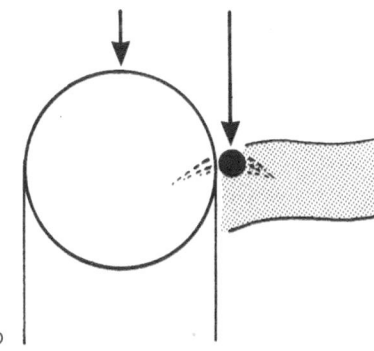

b

Fig. 6.a, b. Artifacts encountered in arthrosonography. **a** Reverberations, **b** hyperbolic artifacts

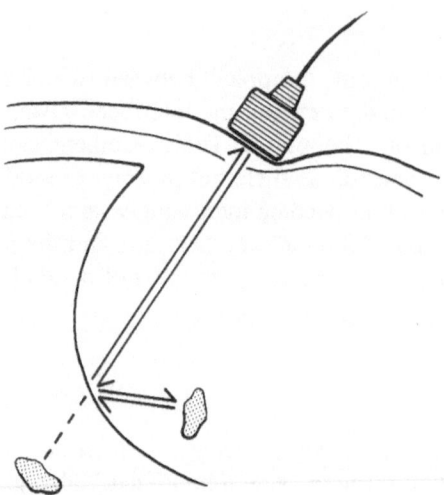

Fig. 7. Acoustic mirror image. The ultrasound instrument cannot recognize the specular effect of the curved, highly reflective interface and portrays the object of interest as a virtual image behind the interface

Acoustic Mirror Image

A curved, intensely echogenic interface between two different media can reflect the ultrasound waves like a mirror, producing a mirror-image type of artifact (Fig. 7). The ultrasound instrument is unable to recognize the "mirror image" as being spurious.

This phenomenon was first observed in the diaphragm, which behaves much like a concave mirror. Hepatic lesions encounterd by the reflected ultrasound beam are displayed as virtual images behind the diaphragm. The acoustic mirror image, first described by Cosgrove, has so far been observed only in upper abdominal ultrasound. It is included here for completeness.

Special Phenomena in Arthrosonography

The curved course of tendons and bones in arthrosonography can lead to special phenomena that must be known so that images can be interpreted correctly.

"Wandering Echo" Phenomenon

Tendons with a curved course appear most echogenic at sites where they are struck at right angles by the ultrasound beam. Other parts of the tendon that are oriented obliquely to the beam appear falsely hypoechoic as a result of diffraction and refraction. The more tangentially a tendon segment is struck by the beam in the static examination, the less echogenic it will appear.

In real-time scanning a bright echo will be seen at the point where the beam is perpendicular to the tendon. This point will "wander" as the beam is moved. This is seen, for example, on longitudinal scans of the ankle and subtaler joints showing the tendons of extensor digitorum longus and in examinations of the supraspinatus tendon at the shoulder during contraction and relaxation of the muscle.

The phenomenon of differing echogenicity from the same structure is new and is of major importance in arthrosonography (Fig. 8 and 9).

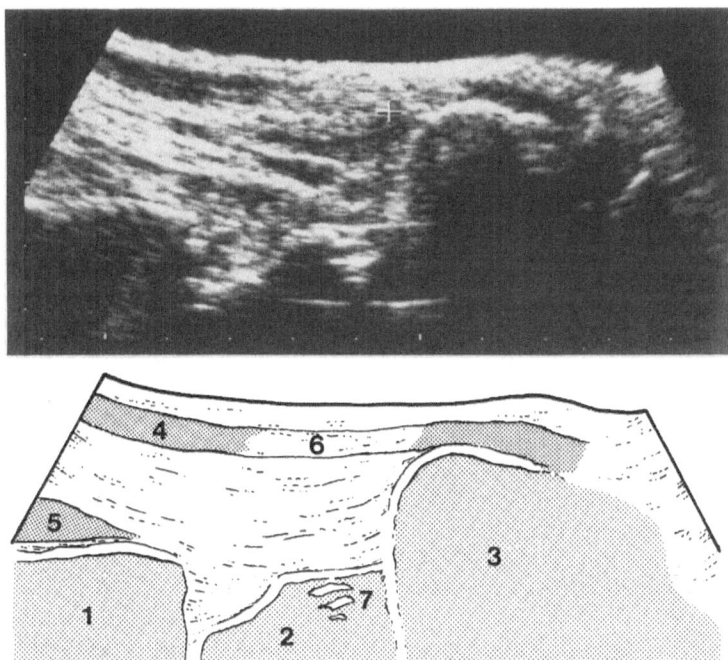

Fig. 8. "Wandering echo" over the Achilles tendon and reverberations on the bone surface, longitudinal scan over the Achilles tendon. **1** Tibia, **2** talus, **3** calcaneus, **4** Achilles tendon, **5** flexor hallucis longus, **6** hyperechoic portion of Achilles tendon (this segment is almost perpendicular to the ultrasound beam), **7** reverberations on the surface of the talus

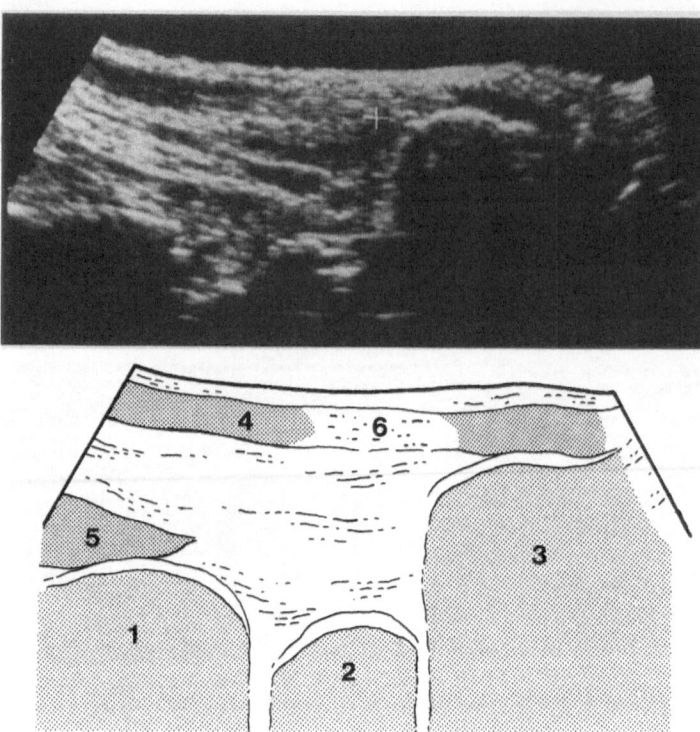

Fig. 9. Wandering echo phenomenon on the Achilles tendon, longitudinal scan. **1** Tibia, **2** talus, **3** calcaneus, **4** Achilles tendon, **5** flexor hallucis longus, **6** hyperechoic tendon segment oriented perpendicular to the beam

Pseudodefect (Fig. 10)

When a curved bony surface is struck almost tangentially by the beam, the absence of echo return from that site can mimic a defect in the bone. This artifact can be identified as such by noting that the beam does not define the "floor" of the defect. The pseudodefect phenomenon is most commonly seen on the lateral and medial surfaces of the distal femoral condyle. It is manifested by an apparent discontinuity in the cortical bone at the junction of the femoral shaft and condyle close to the paraosseous joint pouch when the beam is swept longitudinally over the knee from the posterior side (Fig. 11). The artifact is easily eliminated by redirecting the beam somewhat obliquely into the paraosseous joint pouch. When the beam no longer strikes the site tangentially, the pseudodefect will disappear. The more sound waves impinge on this apparent bony lesion, the more obvious it is that the bone at that location is intact.

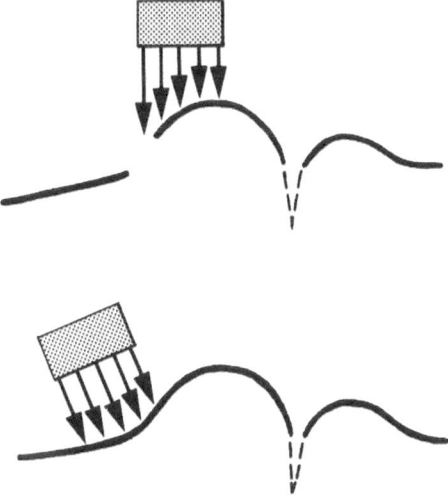

Fig. 10. "Pseudodefect," recognized as such on the lower scan by redirecting the beam

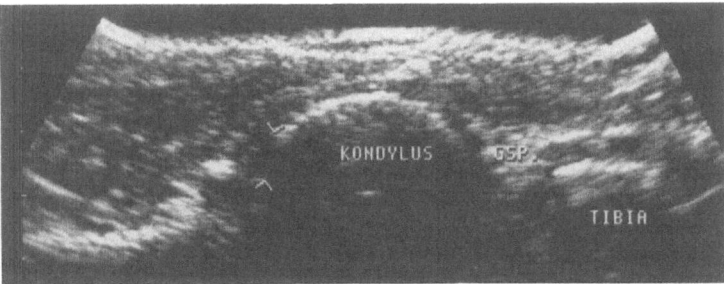

Fig. 11. "Pseudodefect" in the lateral femoral condyle on a posterior longitudinal scan *(arrow heads)*. There is an apparent discontinuity in the cortex where the bone surface is struck tangentially by the beam. *Kondylus:* Condyle

Special Problems in Arthrosonography

1. Only cartilage that is struck by the beam in orthograde fashion (e.g., the cartilage over the condyle) is defined with acceptable clarity.
2. Structures oriented parallel to the beam do not give a satisfactory echo and are not visualized.
3. Bony surfaces cause significant scatter because of their acoustic roughness.
4. Tendons, ligaments, connective tissue, and fat normally do not have sufficient impedance differences to be defined as separate structures, unless contrast is provided by an inflammatory process such as tenosynovitis.

Description of Findings

The written description of ultrasound findings is an important responsibility of the examining physician, who should apply standard nomenclature along with special sonographic terms. It may be helpful to supplement some descriptions with simple drawings. Subjectivity in the reporting of findings can be minimized by using a standard nomenclature and stating the findings as descriptively but as concisely a possible. As in all types of ultrasound examination, particular emphasis is placed upon the following:

- location
- contour
- shape
- structure
- size.

A given finding should be described so fully and uniquely that a subsequent examiner can locate it without difficulty and recognize and changes that have occured.

Because of variations in instrument settings, the echo pattern is the most difficult quality to be described. Since different equipment settings result in different echo characteristics, agreement on standard settings is required. As blood vessels can be visualized around any joint, they provide the best reference objects for making standard instrument settings.

Image Documentation

The documentation of ultrasound findings is essential. Since it is not possible to define scan planes with absolute precision, findings should be documented in such a way that a maximum number of familiar and plainly recognizable landmarks are portrayed.

One way of solving the image documentation problem is by making a video-tape record of the examination. This method has the advantage of documenting the examination in its entirety while also demonstrating articular motion.

The following documentation methods are available:

Documentation of individual sonograms by
- instant-image camera
- video printer
- 35-mm camera
- multiformat camera

Film documentation by
- videotape
- Super-8 movie film.

At present the instant-image camera appears to have been superseded by the video printer, the latter being faster, less costly, and easier to use. A potential disadvantage is that video printouts may not retain their quality as long as Polaroid pictures, but this has yet to be determined.

The 35-mm camera continues to be an interesting alternative. The image quality is high, but transferring the image to paper with a photographic enlarger is costly and time consuming.

Videotape recorders have largely replaced movie cameras because they are cheaper and allow immediate playback. They play a major role in the documentation of articular examinations with ultrasound. At present, the combined use of a videotape recorder and video printer appears to be ideal for the documentation of findings.

A final alternative is the multiformat camera, which utilizes X-ray film sheets. An X-ray developing machine must be available for processing.

As in other applications of diagnostic ultrasound, the examiner should first make a complete description of the arthrosonographic findings before attempting to make a definitive evaluation in the light of clinical data and other information.

It is advantageous to select instrument settings like those conventionally used for the upper abdomen and other familiar areas. This means that blood vessels should appear hypoechoic to echo-free. The standard white-on-black format is recommended for ease of visual interpretation.

Shoulder Joint

Technique of Examination

Because the soulder joint is stabilized essentially by muscles rather than by the geometric shape of the joint surfaces, many lesions of the soft-tissue envelope can produce a muscular imbalance leading to dysfunction. The shoulder joint is easily accessible from several sides, making it an excellent object for sonographic evaluation.

Five and 7.5-MHz transducers are suitable for examinations of the shoulder. The use of a standoff pad is recommended, as otherwise contact between the probe and skin may be lost in certain projections, especially in thin patients. Also, a standoff pad will place immediate subcutaneous tissues within the optimum focal zone of the transducer.

For the examination the patient is seated on a stool between the examiner and the ultrasound unit or monitor. The examination is performed with the arm adducted to the thorax and the elbow flexed 90° (Fig. 12). The examiner controls the transducer with one hand while holding the patient's forearm with the other hand. For transverse scans the examiner can rotate the upper arm and hold the transducer steady to bring adjacent areas of the proximal humerus and surrouding soft tissues beneath the probe. Motion sequences can be observed and repeated as required. The examination begins by locating and identifying key anatomic landmarks. For this the soulder is scanned on multiple planes. We recommend scanning two mutually perpendicular planes each on the posterior, lateral, and anterior aspects of the joint. The structures are evaluated for sonographic changes. It is best to proceed systematically, e. g., by starting posteriorly and moving the transducer over the lateral to the anterior aspect of the shoulder while visualizing the desired planes.

Scan planes should be established with reference to bony landmarks to facilitate rapid orientation, and comparable findings can be documented.

The second phase of the ultrasound examination consists of function testing. Pressure is applied to the posterior aspect of the upper arm to test the posterioanterior stability of the joint, and anteroposterior stability is assessed by pulling the upper arm backward. On the lateral longitudinal scan, the arm is abducted to determine whether large calcifications or bony lesions of the greater tuberosity are gliding beneath or impinging on the acromion, thereby limiting further abduction. The retroversion angle of the humeral head is determined with the patient supine. A transducer with attached spirit level is used to establish a true horizontal.

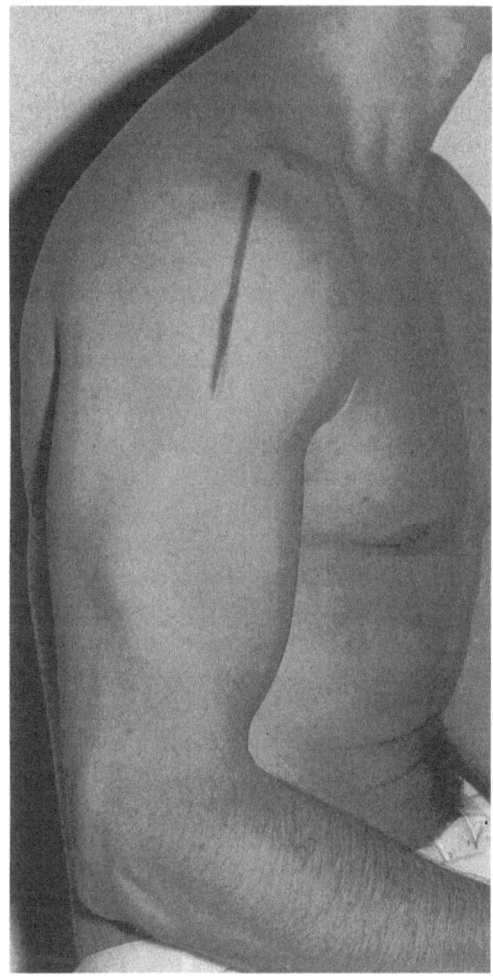

Fig. 12. Position for arthrosonography of the shoulder. The upper arm is adducted to the thorax, and the elbow is flexed to 90°. The examination proceeds from the posterior to the anterior side

An anterior transverse scan is taken over the proximal humerus, and the upper arm is rotated until the intertubercular sulcus is directed vertically. With the arm held in that position, an anterior scan is performed at the level of the trochlea of the humerus. The retroversion angle can be determined from both scans.

Normal Sonographic Anatomy

The anatomy of the shoulder joint is defined from the posterior, lateral, and anterior aspects on mutually perpendicular planes. The principal anatomic structures are listed below.

1. Acromion
2. Coracoid
3. Clavicle
4. Humerus
5. Greater tuberosity
6. Lesser tuberosity
7. Scapula

8. Long biceps tendon
9. Deltoid muscle
10. Infraspinatus muscle
11. Teres minor muscle
12. Supraspinatus muscle
13. Supraspinatus tendon
14. Subscapularis muscle

These structures may be cut longitudinally or transversely by the ultrasound beam, depending on the position of the image plane. The essential landmarks are the bones of the shoulder joint, which should be imaged consistently in the same or comparable views. Standard imaging planes have several advantages, including rapid orientation for the examiner and availability of findings that can be easily compared and reviewed. The position of the scans relative to the body surface, the corresponding anatomic sections, and the sonographic appearance of the anatomic structures are illustrated in Figs. 13–20.

The planes illustrated provide virtually complete coverage of the shoulder joint. Because two mutually perpendicular views are obtained on the posterior, lateral, and anterior sides, artifacts are easily recognized.

The scapulohumeral joint is examined on six planes of section. The acromioclavicular joint, an important subsidiary joint of the shoulder, is visualized on a nearly coronal plane and is evaluated for injury or degenerative change.

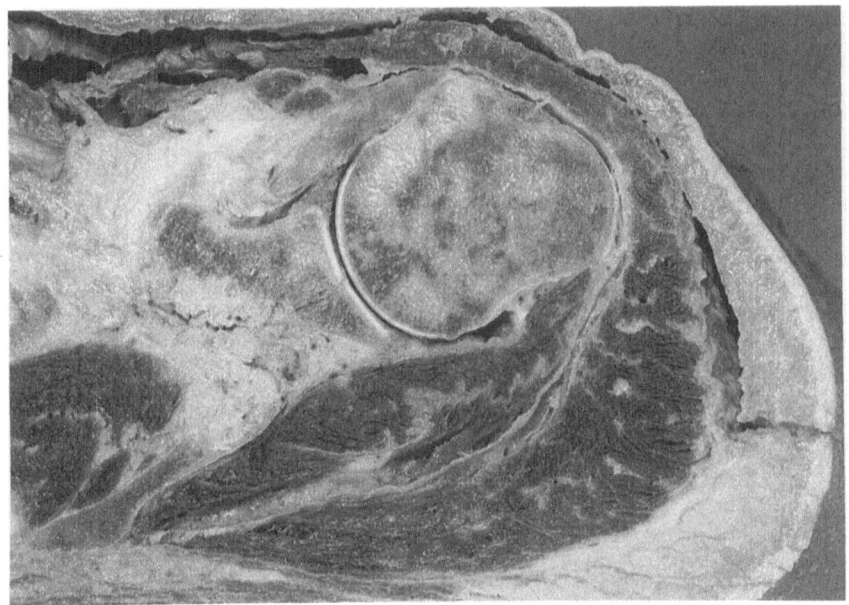

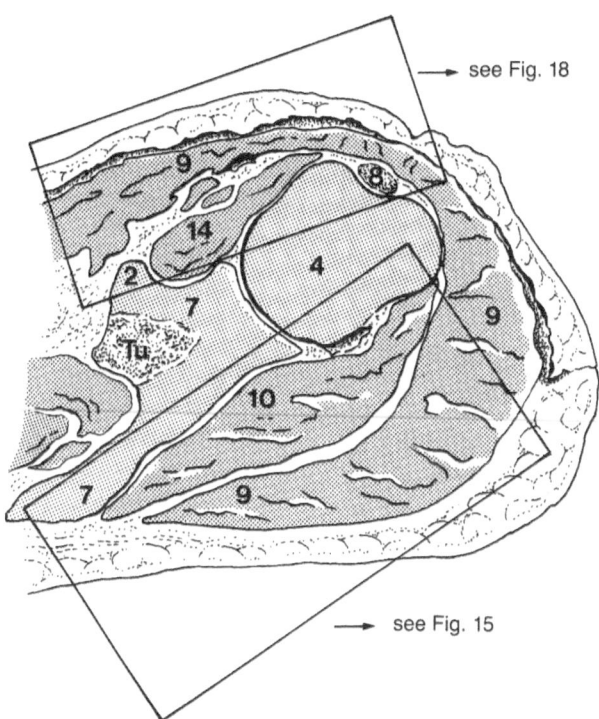

see Fig. 18

see Fig. 15

Fig. 13. Anatomic transverse section through a right shoulder. There is metastatic tumor (Tu) in the scapula. **2** Coracoid process, **4** proximal humerus, **7** scapula, **8** long biceps tendon in intertubercular sulcus, **9** deltoid muscle, **10** infraspinatus muscle, **14** subscapularis muscle

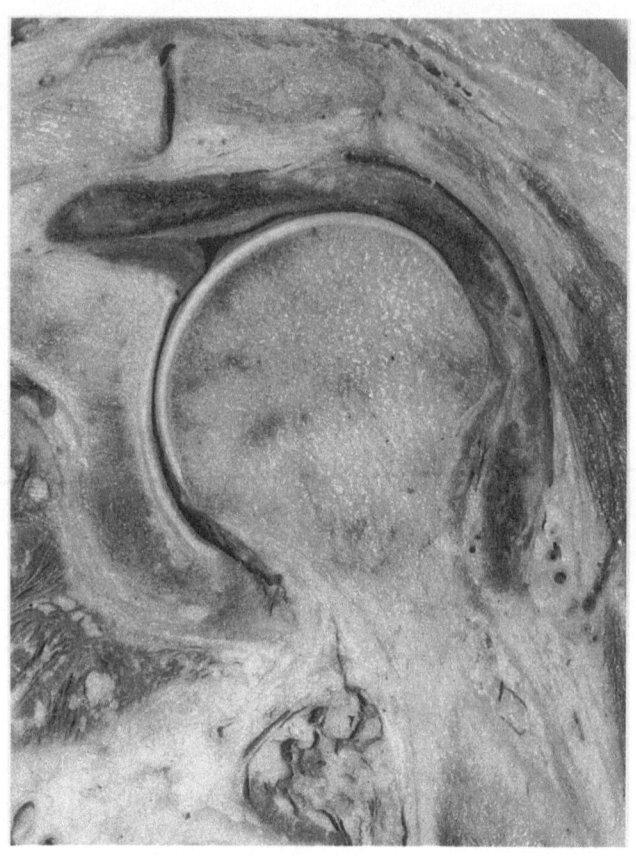

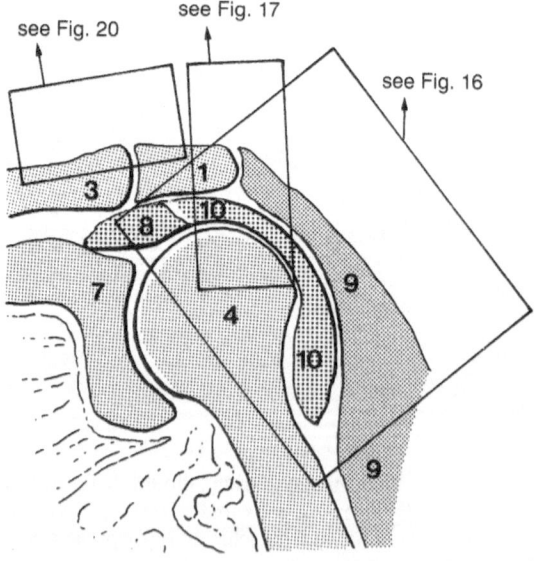

see Fig. 20

see Fig. 17

see Fig. 16

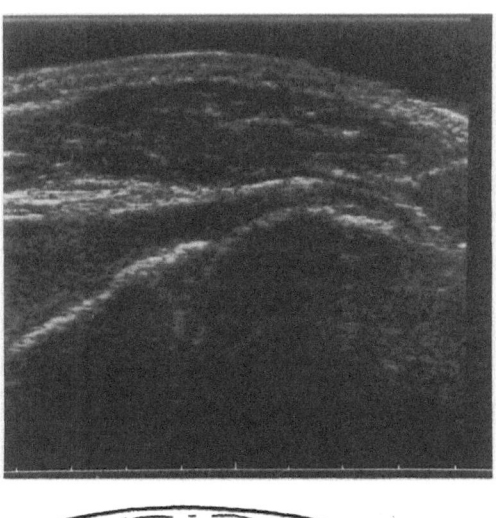

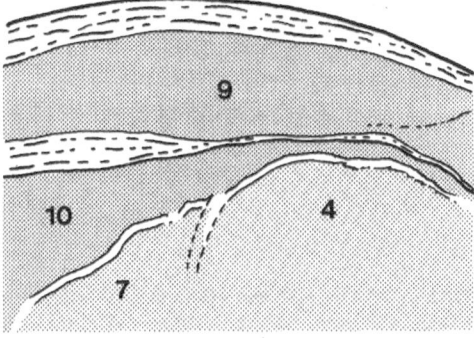

Fig. 15. Posterior transverse scan in the infraspinous fossa. Anatomic relationships are shown in Fig. 13 *(bottom half)*. **4** Proximal humerus, **7** scapula, **9** deltoid muscle (cut transversely), **10** infraspinatus muscle (cut longitudinally)

Fig. 14. Anatomic coronal section through the right shoulder. **1** Acromion, **3** acromial end of clavicle, **4** proximal humerus, **7** scapula, **8** long biceps tendon, **9** deltoid muscle, **10** external rotators

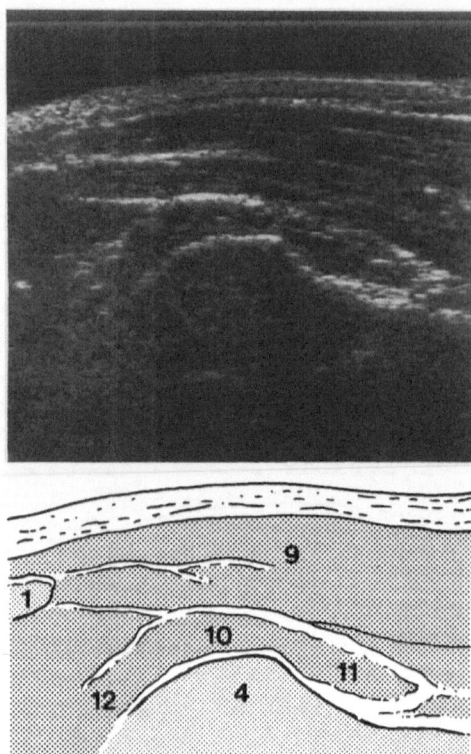

Fig. 16. Posterior longitudinal scan. With the upper arm in internal rotation, this posterior scan cuts transversely the muscular portion of the external rotators (teres minor, infraspinatus, supraspinatus; see Fig. 14). **1** Acromion, **4** humerus, **9** deltoid muscle (cut longitudinally), **10** infraspinatus muscle, **11** teres minor muscle, **12** supraspinatus muscle

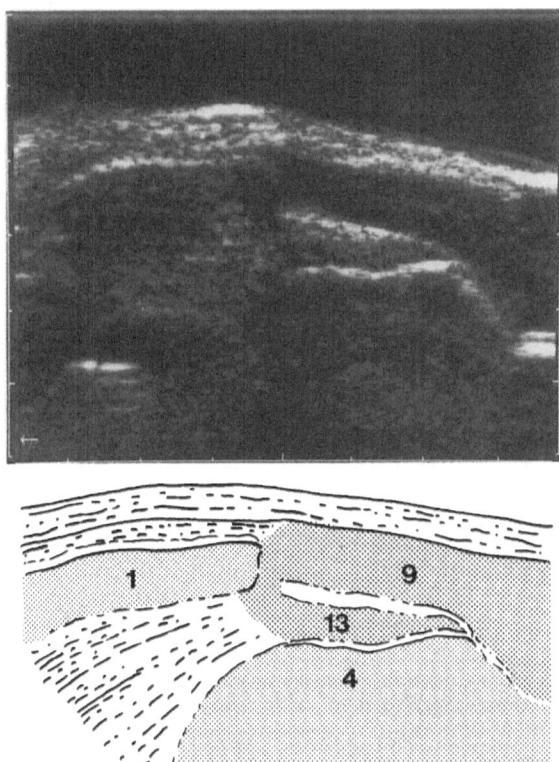

Fig. 17. Coronal scan demonstrating the supraspinatus tendon (see Fig. 14). **1** Acromion, **4** proximal humerus, **9** deltoid muscle (cut longitudinally), **13** supraspinatus tendon

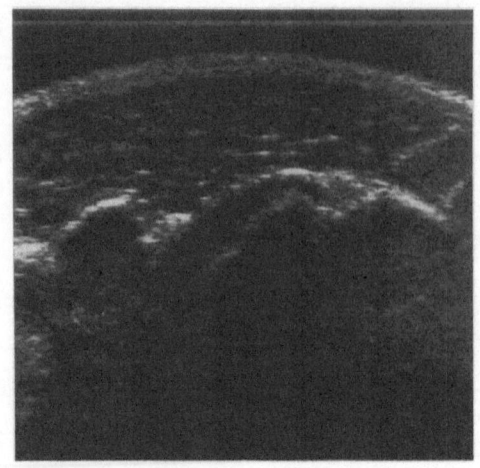

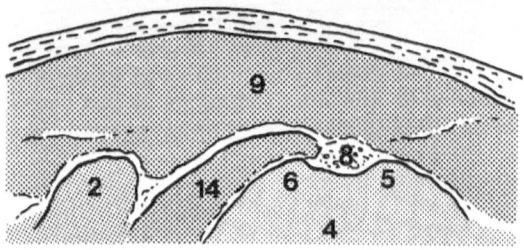

Fig. 18. Anterior transverse scan (see top half of Fig. 13). **2** Coracoid process, **4** proximal humerus, **5** greater tuberosity, **6** lesser tuberosity, **8** long biceps tendon (cut transversely in the intertubercular sulcus), **9** deltoid muscle (cut transversely), **14** subscapularis muscle

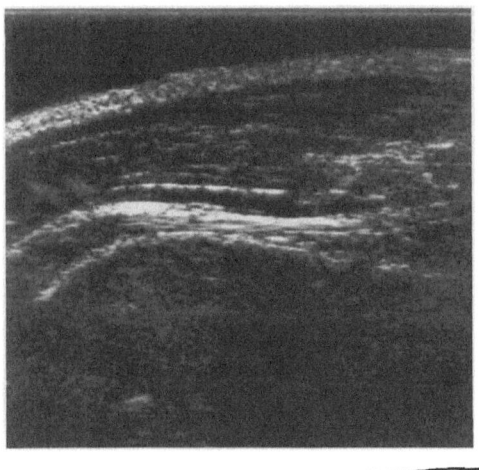

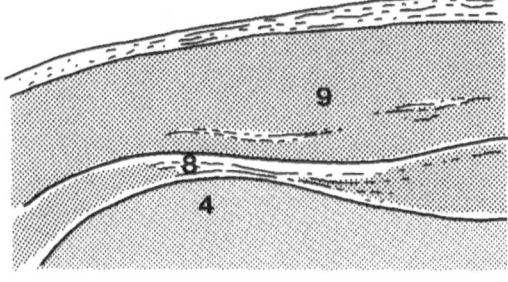

Fig. 19. Anterior longitudinal scan demonstrating the long biceps tendon in the intertubercular sulcus. **4** Proximal humerus, **8** long biceps tendon (cut longitudinally), **9** deltoid muscle (cut longitudinally)

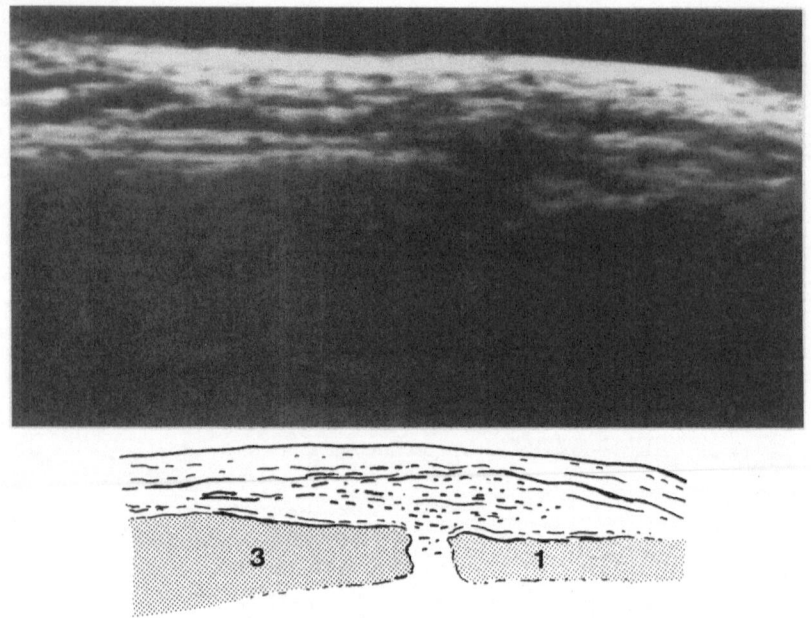

Fig. 20. Scan over the acromioclavicular joint (see Fig. 14). **1** Acromion, **3** acromial end of clavicle

Interpretive Criteria

The scans should be evaluated for
- osseous changes,
- changes in the joint cavity and bursae,
- soft-tissue changes,
- decreased motion or stability, and (if necessary)
- measurement of retroversion.

Osseous changes present as discontinuities in the outer contour of the cortical bone. They may result from neoplastic disease, bony avulsion of the supraspinatus tendon, rheumatoid disease (Fig. 21), or a Hill-Sachs lesion following dislocation of the shoulder (Fig. 22). Fractures may result in a stepoff deformity that interferes with normal joint motion (Fig. 23). In degenerative arthritis, osteophytes can form at the junction of the humeral head and greater tuberosity at the level of the anatomic neck.

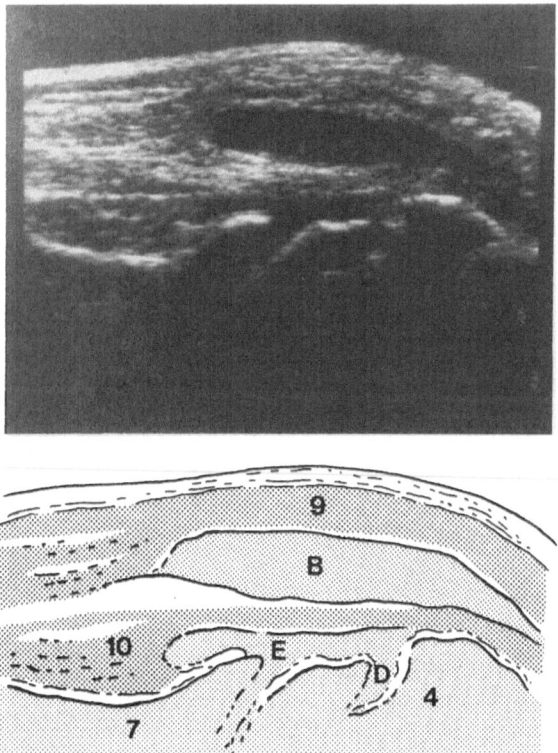

Fig. 21. Shoulder joint involvement in rheumatioid arthritis. Posterior transverse scan. The posterior contour of the proximal humerus is interrupted by a defect (**D**), and the joint capsule is distended by effusion (**E**). There is an additional fluid collection in the subdeltoid bursa (**B**). **4** Proximal humerus, **7** scapula, **9** deltoid muscle, **10** infraspinatus muscle

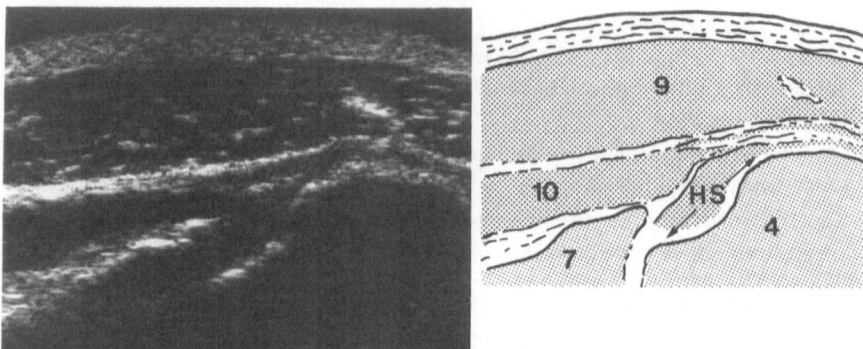

Fig. 22. Habitual dislocation of the right shoulder. Posterior transverse scan. The Hill-Sachs lesion (**HS**) enters the glenoid fossa as the upper arm is rotated externally. **4** Proximal humerus, **7** scapula, **9** deltoid muscle, **10** infraspinatus muscle

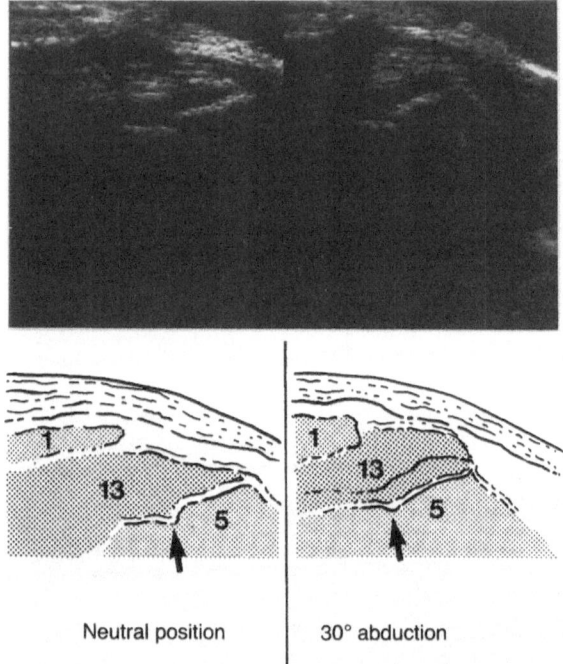

Neutral position | 30° abduction

Fig. 23. Malunion following an avulsion fracture of the greater tuberosity during shoulder dislocation. Coronal scan. The malunited avulsion fracture of the greater tuberosity (**5**) has created a step in the cranial contour of the proximal humerus (**arrow**). On abduction of the upper arm *(right half of figure)* the supraspinatus tendon (**13**) becomes incarcerated between the greater tuberosity and acromion (**1**), preventing further abduction at the humeroscapular joint

Changes in the joint cavity are best appreciated on posterior scans and generally consist of distension of the joint capsule by effusion. Of the various articular recesses (axillary, subscapular, long biceps tendon), only the recess of the long biceps tendon (see Fig. 25) can be evaluated. This recess fills with fluid when there is intra-articular effusion, the effusion of rheumatoid disease often containing internal echoes as a result of fibrin deposition.

Changes in the bursae frequently coexist with joint effusions. The major causes are diseases of the rheumatoid series. Effusions may also accompany dislocation or other types of injury.

The subdeltoid bursa is diverse in its sonographic morphology. It may extend anteriorly to the intertubercular sulcus and posteriorly onto the scapula (Fig. 24). It is continuous superiorly with the subacromial bursa. When there is effusion in the subacromial bursa but no fluid in the subdeltoid bursa, a triangular space appears between the inferior border of the deltoid muscle and the supraspinatus tendon. This space is plainly visible on the lateral longitudinal scan.

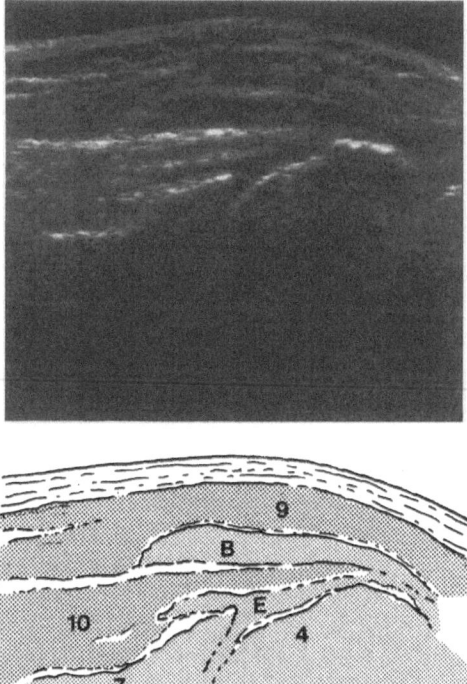

Fig. 24. Shoulder joint involvement in rheumatoid arthritis. Posterior transverse scan. The arthritis has resulted in joint effusion (**E**) and distension of the subdeltoid bursa (**B**). The posterior contour of the proximal humerus is free of defects. **4** Proximal humerus, **7** scapula, **9** deltoid muscle, **10** infraspinatus muscle

The coracobrachial bursa is demonstrated anteriorly on transverse and longitudinal scans. It directly overlies the subscapularis muscle and extends laterally from the coracoid, in some cases reaching the intertubercular sulcus. On longitudinal scans one should watch for a narrow, hypoechoic structure (representing the joint capsule) interposed between the long biceps tendon and the bursa. This structure can be used to differentiate effusion in the recess of the long biceps tendon (Fig. 25) from coracobrachial bursitis (Fig. 26) on the anterior longitudinal scan. Rheumatoid diseases are the most common cause of a distended coracobrachial bursa. Other causes include injuries of the subscapularis muscle and shoulder joint effusions in general, since the coracobrachial bursa frequently communicates with the joint.

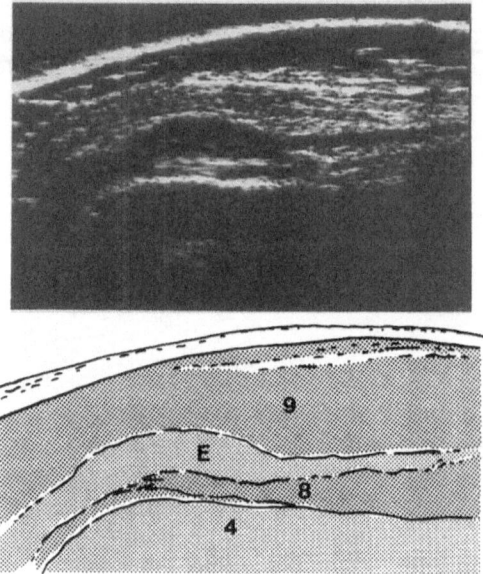

Fig. 25. Shoulder joint involvement in rheumatoid arthritis. Anterior longitudinal scan. The shoulder joint effusion (**E**) fills the recess of the long biceps tendon. **4** Proximal humerus, **8** long biceps tendon, **9** deltoid muscle. (See also Fig. 26 concerning identification of the long biceps tendon and effusion in the coracobrachial bursa)

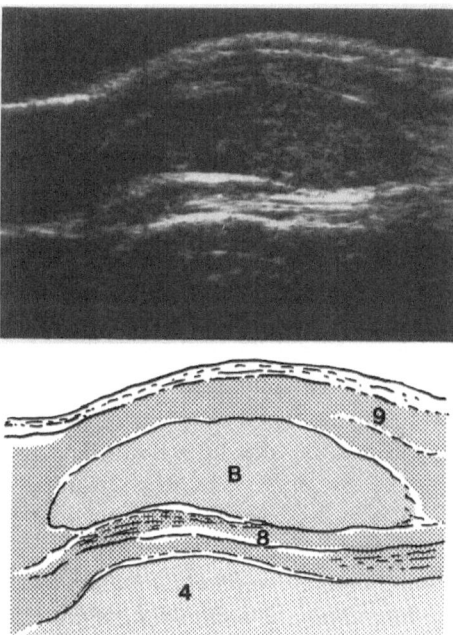

Fig. 26. Shoulder joint involvement in rheumatoid arthritis. Anterior longitudinal scan. There is no significant joint effusion. The coracobrachial bursa (**B**) is expanded by hypoechoic material with internal echoes. The bursa is separated from the recess of the long biceps tendon by an echogenic layer of connective tissue (see also Fig. 25). **4** Proximal humerus, **8** long biceps tendon, **9** deltoid muscle

Soft-tissue changes involve the muscles and tendons of the shoulder joint. Trauma may completely disrupt the continuity of these structures or may cause a bony tendon avulsion with displacement of the avulsed fragment. Fresh musculotendinous ruptures are usually accompanied by bloody effusions which spread into adjacent bursae and within the joint (see Fig. 39). Even old rotator cuff tears can incite effusion as a result of disordered joint function. Degenerative soft-tissue changes generally involve the tendinous portions of the muscles, the supraspinatus tendon being the most commonly affected. Ultrasound shows an echogenic area surrounded by a hypoechoic zone separating it from the normally echogenic tendon tissue (see Fig. 31). With large foci of degenerative change, the hypoechoic zone may traverse the entire cross-section of the tendon.

Stability testing should be performed in both shoulders so that the results for each side can be compared, and the degree of displacement should be assessed in the light of clinical complaints (Fig. 27). The range of individual variation is substantial, since the mobility of the shoulder joint tends to match the patient's constitutional level of joint mobility. Thus, a displacement of 5 mm is not pathologic in individuals with weak connective tissues and ligamentous laxity, but an equal displacement may have pathologic significance in patients with tight connective tissues, especially when there is subjective shoulder instability or a coexisting soft-tissue injury.

Sonography is excellent for function testing owing to its ability to monitor soft-tissue movements in real time. Thus, the posterior transverse scan can be performed to determine whether a Hill-Sachs defect engages the glenoid rim on external rotation of the arm and might cause the humeral head to dislocate anteriorly when subsequent internal rotation is performed.

An avulsion fracture of the greater tuberosity creates a stepoff deformity in the proximal humerus which may impinge on the acromion during abduction and block further extension of the arm (see Fig. 23).

Measurement of the retroversion angle of the humeral head is indicated when planning the operative treatment of a shoulder dislocation or as a prelude to the corrective osteotomy of a malunited fracture (see Fig. 41).

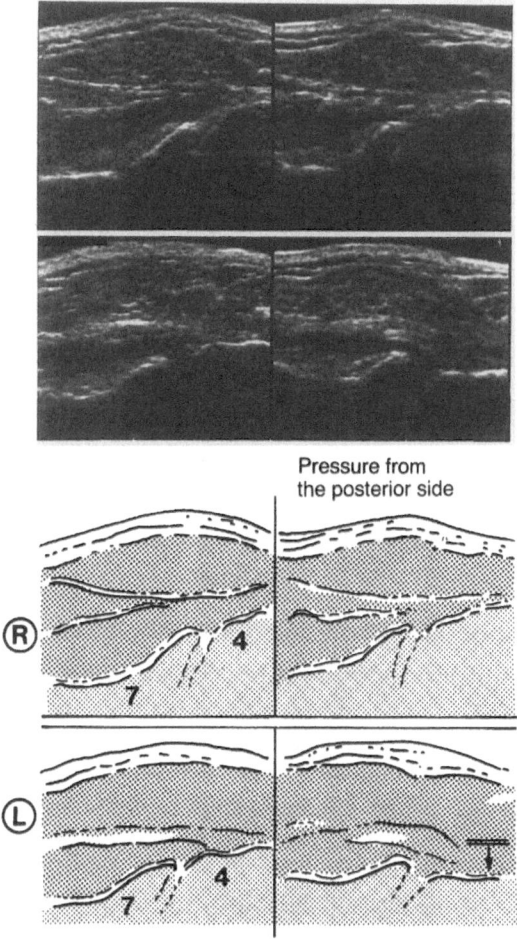

Fig. 27. Instability of the left shoulder secondary to an extensive rotator cuff tear. Functional views in the posterior transverse projection. In the injured left shoulder *(bottom half of figure)*, pressure from the posterior side *(arrow)* displaces the proximal humerus (4) forward. Equal pressure on the uninjured right side, shown for comparison, does not cause significant displacement. **4** Proximal humerus, **7** scapula

Pathologic Conditions

Rheumatoid Arthritis (see Figs. 21, 24–26)

Rheumatoid arthritis of the shoulder produces changes characterized by osseous defects and inflammatory proliferative synovitis (joint effusion, bursitis). Osseous defects are most commonly detected on anterior and posterior scans. Biplane imaging is especially important on the posterior side, where a prominent anatomic neck can simulate a defect. Isolated shoulder arthritis with no involvement of the bursae leads to distension of the posterior capsule and the recess of the long biceps tendon. The coracobrachial bursa will also become distended if the latter communicates with the joint. The subdeltoid bursa may extend far posteriorly onto the scapula.

Supraspinatus Syndrome (Figs. 28–31)

The lateral longitudinal scan displays the supraspinatus tendon as a triangular echogenic structure overlying the proximal humerus. Rotation of the arm will bring successive portions of the tendon beneath the probe, allowing them to be examined with a perpendicular beam incidence.

On the lateral transverse scan and in scans over the "coracoacromial window," the supraspinatus tendon shows varying echo characteristics due to its curved course along the proximal humerus. The part of the tendon nearst the transducer and perpendicular to it appears hyperechoic, while the adjacent portions present an increasingly oblique surface to the transducer and appear correspondingly hypoechoic. Evaluation of the supraspinatus tendon for structural changes is made difficult by this "arc effect." (Hence the lateral transverse scan is not included among the standard views and is used only to check findings noted on the coronal views.)

The hypoechoic zones bordering large degenerative foci have the same sonographic appearance as the hypoechoic bands of full-thickness rotator cuff tears without retraction (see Fig. 32). However, hyperechoic calcifications commonly occur in large areas of degenrative change, and the associated acoustic shadow on the proximal humerus will serve to distinguish the lesion from a rotator cuff tear.

With advancing age, degenerative changes are increasingly likely to be found in the distal portion of the supraspinatus tendon. These changes present sonographically as highly echogenic areas with hypoechoic borders. Calcium-rich areas of degenerative change cast an acoustic shadow (Figs. 28 and 29).

Acoustic shadowing by large, sonodense structural changes interrupts the outer contour of the humerus (Fig. 29).

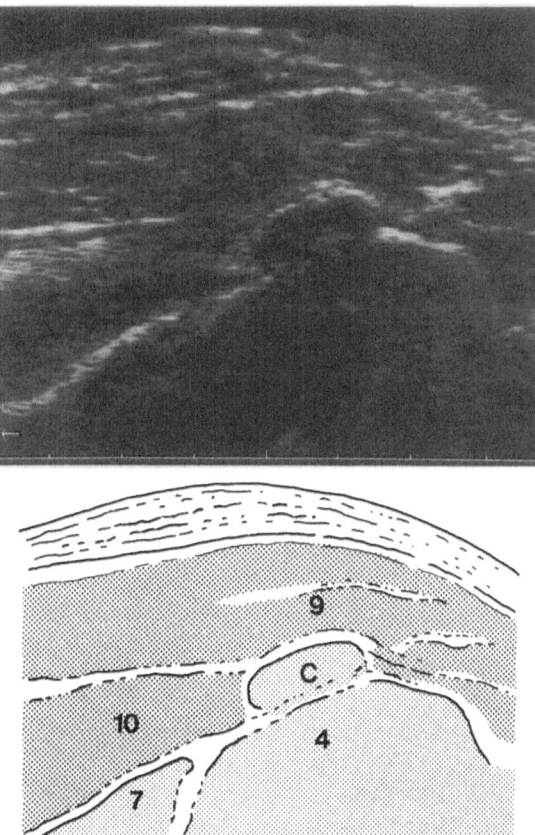

Fig. 28. Supraspinatus syndrome. Posterior transverse scan shows multiple calcifications in the external rotators (see Fig. 30). The calcification (**C**) in the infraspinatus muscle (**10**) casts a shadow on the underlying posterior contour of the proximal humerus (**4**). **7** Scapula, **9** deltoid muscle

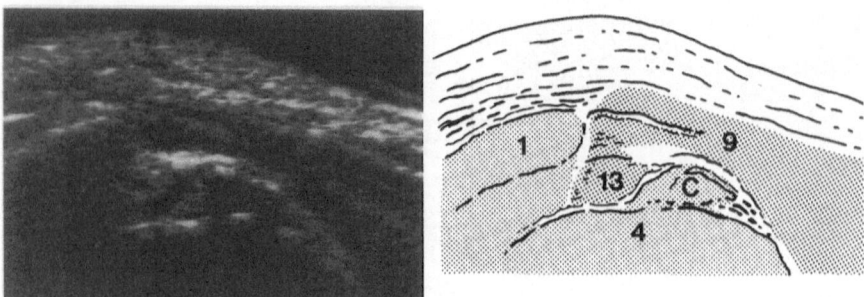

Fig. 29. Same patient as in Fig. 28, coronal scan. The large calcification (C) in the supraspinatus tendon (13) casts a shadow on the underlying cranial contour of the proximal humerus (4). The hypoechoic area medial to the calcification should not be mistaken for a rotator cuff tear (see Fig. 32). 1 Acromion, 9 deltoid muscle

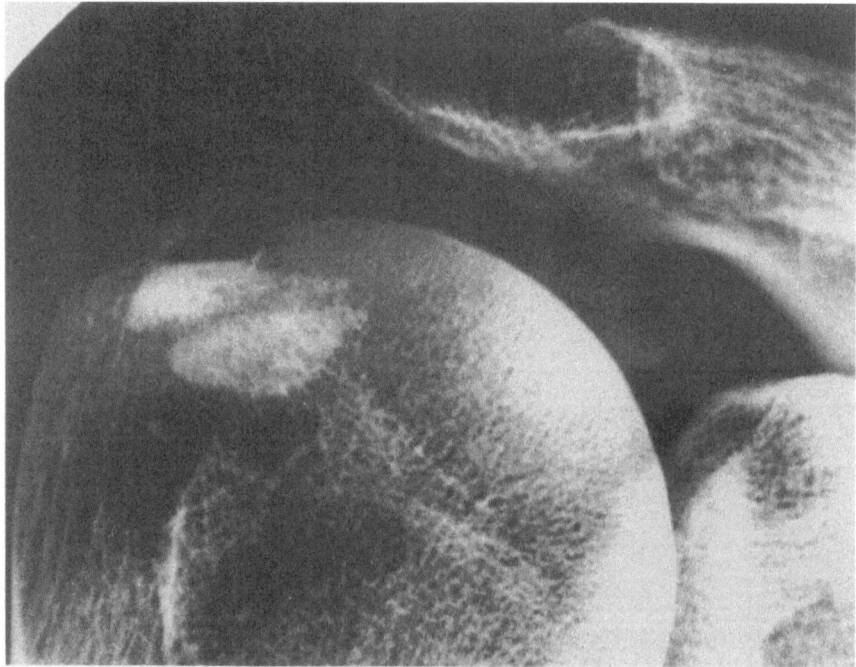

Fig. 30. Roentgenogram of the patient in Figs. 28 and 29. The calcifications form a string-of-beads pattern in the external rotators. The supraspinatus tendon and infraspinatus muscle are affected

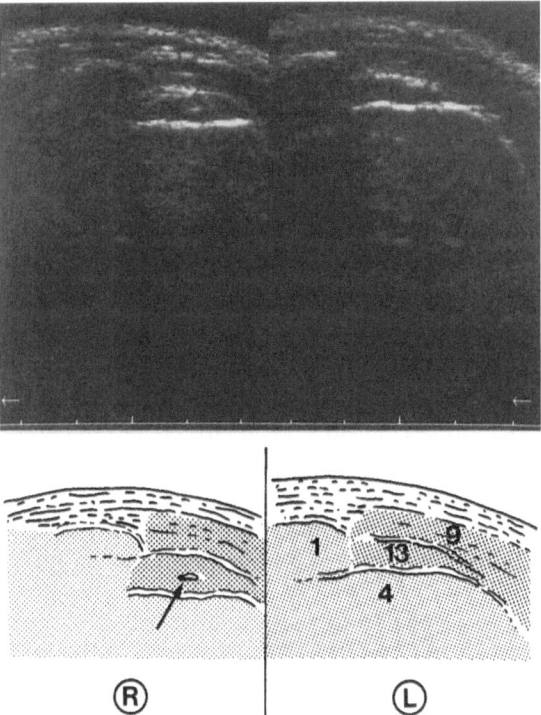

Fig. 31. Supraspinatus syndrome. Coronal scan. There is an echogenic structural abnormality (**arrow**) surrounded by a hypoechoic zone in the supraspinatus tendon (**13**) on the affected right side. The lesion does not cast a shadow on the upper contour of the humerus. The unaffected left side is shown for comparison. **1** Acromion, **4** proximal humerus, **9** deltoid muscle, **13** supraspinatus tendon

Rotator Cuff Tears (Figs. 32-38)

Full-thickness cuff tears with retraction create a structural discontinuity in the rotator muscles. According to Mack, complete tears with a defect larger than 3 cm can be diagnosed sonographically with a confidence level comparable to that of arthrography. Most of these tears are superimposed on a degenerative lesion and occur just lateral to the greater tuberosity of the humerus. With complete avulsion of the external rotators, the changes extend into the posterior image sections. Scans on multiple planes will provide a good spatial impression of the extent of the tear (Figs. 34-38). Complete ruptures may be accompanied by sonograhic changes other than discontinuity. For example, there may be joint effusion distending the posterior part of the capsule or the recess of the long biceps tendon. Because the tear permits the effusion to enter the bursae, the coracobrachial or subdeltoid bursa also is generally visualized.

Incomplete tears and small tears without retraction are more difficult to detect with ultrasound (see Fig. 32). They appear as narrow bands traversing the normal structure of the supraspinatus tendon and cannot always be clearly differentiated from the sonolucencies surrounding large degenerative foci (see Fig. 29).

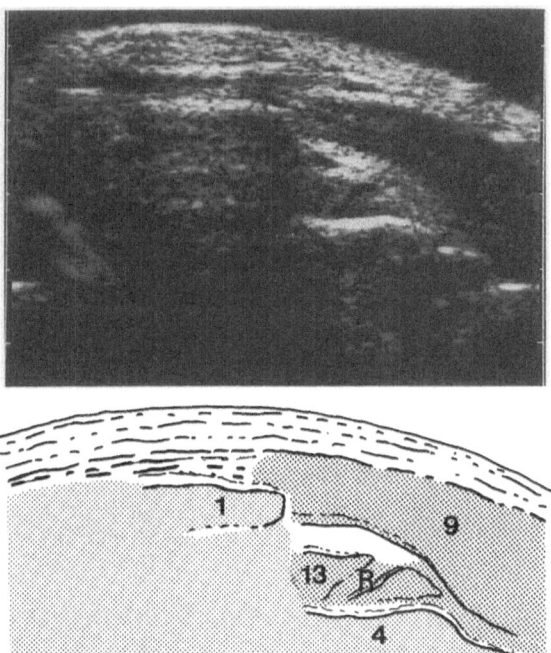

Fig. 32. Rotator cuff tear without retraction. Coronal scan. The echogenic supraspinatus tendon (**13**) is traversed by a hypoechoic band (**R**) representing a rupture of the supraspinatus tendon (see also Fig. 36). Similar hypoechoic bands occur at the periphery of large calcifications (see Fig. 29). Differentiation is aided by noting the cranial contour of the proximal humerus, which is usually obscured by shadow in the presence of large degenerative calcifications; no such shadowing is seen with cuff tears. **1** Acromion, **4** proximal humerus, **9** deltoid muscle

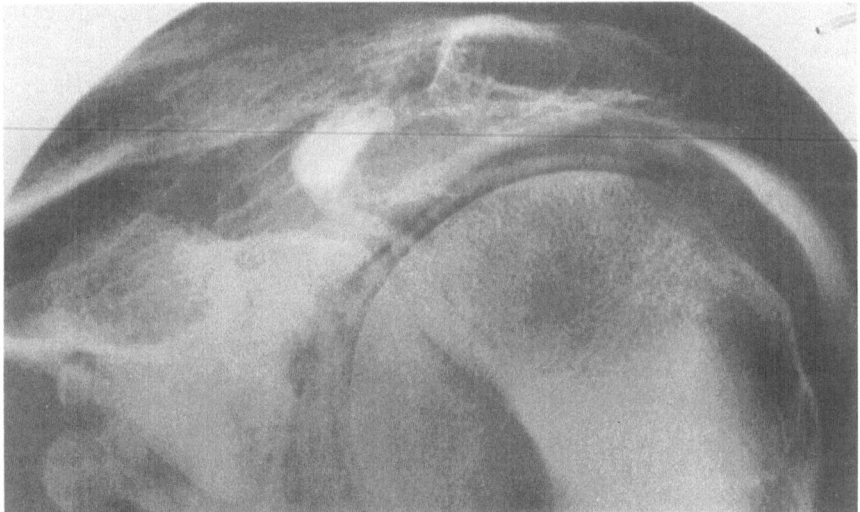

Fig. 33. Arthrogram of the shoulder joint in a rotator cuff tear without retraction. Same patient as in Fig. 32

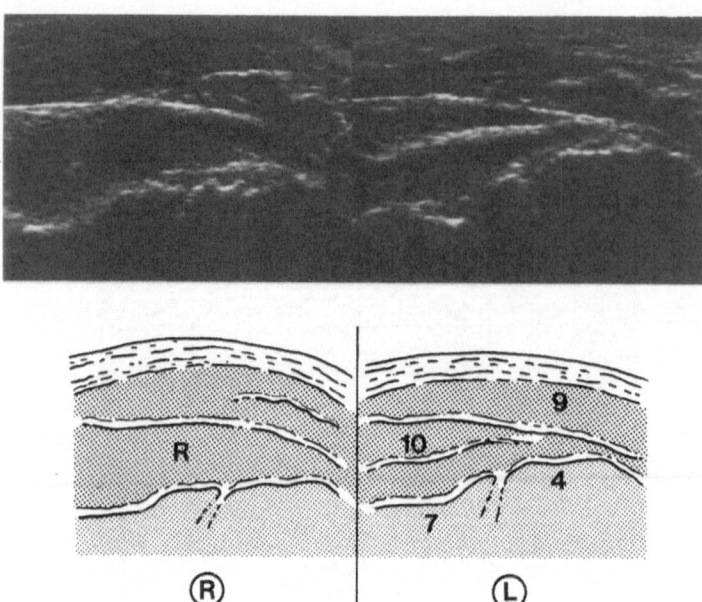

Fig. 34. Rotator cuff tear with retraction. Posterior transverse scan. There is a large rupture of the external rotators affecting the supraspinatus muscle (see Fig. 36) and infraspinatus muscle. Ultrasound shows a marked structural discontinuity in the infraspinatus muscle (**R**) in the affected right shoulder. The healthy left side is shown for comparison. There the muscle retains its normal echo pattern and longitudinal septation (**10**). **4** Proximal humerus, **7** scapula, **9** deltoid muscle

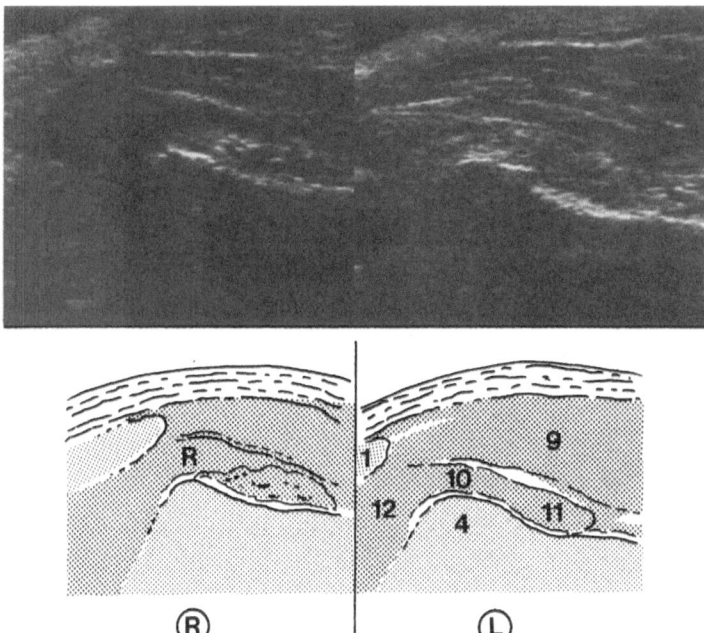

Fig. 35. Same patient as in Fig. 34. Posterior longitudinal scan. This view of the muscular portion of the external rotators demonstrates the extent of the rotator cuff tear. On the injured right side the echo pattern of the muscular portion of the supraspinatus and infraspinatus is obliterated by the tear (**R**). The healthy left side is shown for comparison.
1 Acromion, **4** proximal humerus, **9** deltoid muscle, **10** infraspinatus muscle, **11** teres minor muscle, **12** supraspinatus muscle

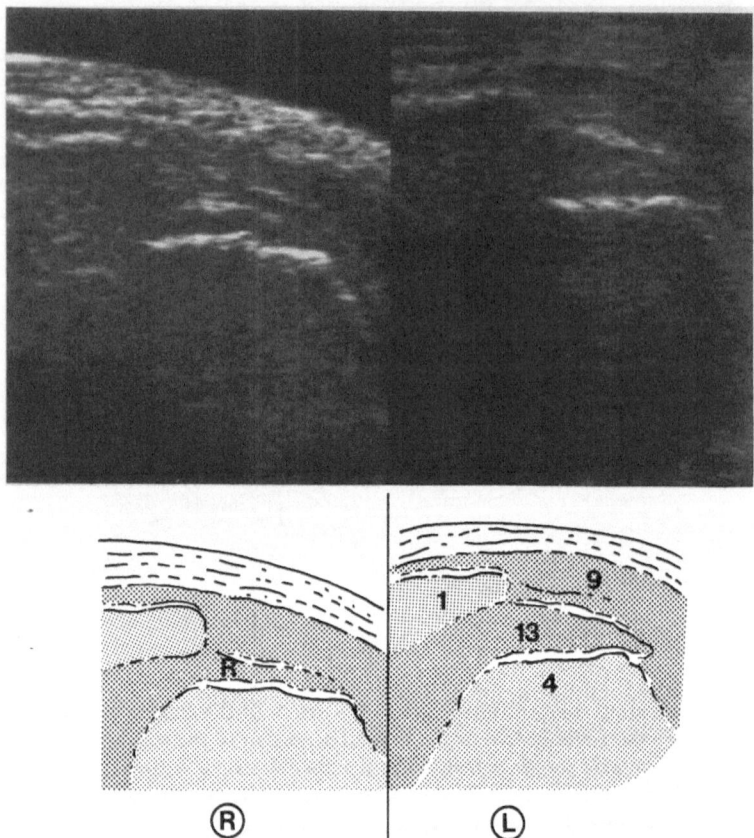

Fig. 36. Same patient as in Fig. 35. Coronal scan shows the deltoid muscle directly over-lying the proximal humerus on the injured right side because of the rotator tear (**R**). The echogenic structure of the supraspinatus tendon is notably absent on this scan. The unin-jured left side is shown for comparison. **1** Acromion, **4** proximal humerus, **9** deltoid muscle, **13** supraspinatus tendon

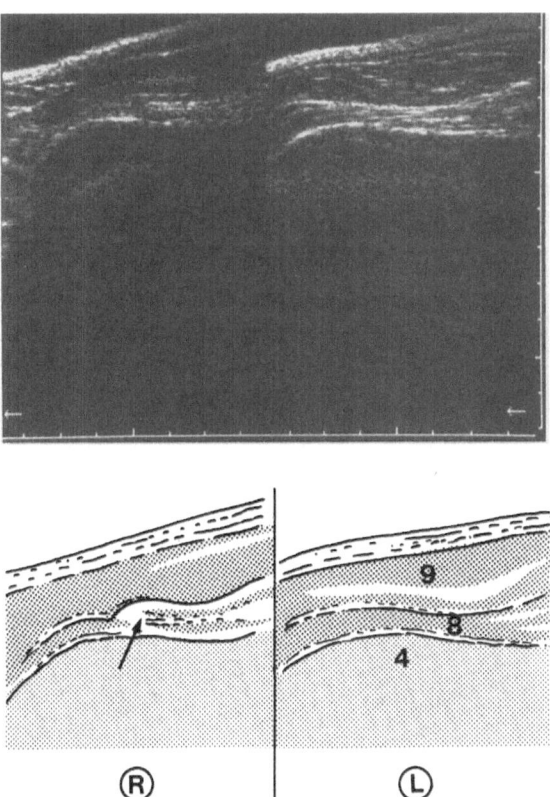

Fig. 37. Old full-thickness rotator cuff tear with retraction (subscapularis muscle and external rotators are not visualized) with concomitant rupture of the long biceps tendon. Anterior longitudinal scan. The stump of the long biceps tendon (**arrow**) on the injured right side is retracted in the recess. The uninjured left side is shown for comparison. (Other injured structures are shown in Fig. 38.) **4** Proximal humerus, **8** long biceps tendon, **9** deltoid muscle

With avulsion of the subscapularis muscle, the structure of the muscle is not visualized on the anterior transverse scan (Fig.38). The deltoid muscle is continuous to the humerus or, in the case of a fresh injury, is separated from it by effusion. Tears of the subscapularis muscle can destabilize the guidance of the long biceps tendon in the intertubercular sulcus. The anterior longitudinal scan over the sulcus is helpful in determining whether the long biceps tendon is displaced or ruptured (see Fig.37).

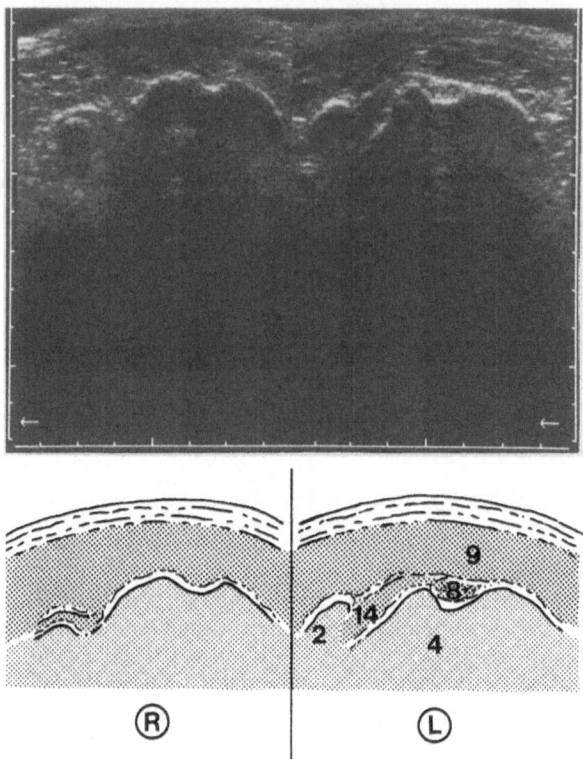

Fig.38. Same patient as in Fig.37. Anterior transverse scan. The structure of the subscapularis muscle (**14**) is absent on the injured right side, and the long biceps tendon is absent from the intertubercular sulcus so that the deltoid fibers directly overlie the anterior aspect of the proximal humerus. The healthy left side is shown for comparison. **2** Coracoid process, **4** proximal humerus, **8** long biceps tendon, **9** deltoid muscle

Rupture of the Long Biceps Tendon (Fig. 39, see also Fig. 37)

This injury is readily diagnosed from clinical signs. Sonography reveals a discontinuity of the tendon in the proximal part of the intertubercular sulcus. The tendon is frayed in the area of the rupture and shows an alternation of hypo- and hyperechoic zones. Fresh injuries may be accompanied by joint effusion, producing enlargement of the recess of the long biceps tendon (Fig. 39). In longstanding ruptures the wall of the recess is generally adherent to the tendon (see Fig. 37).

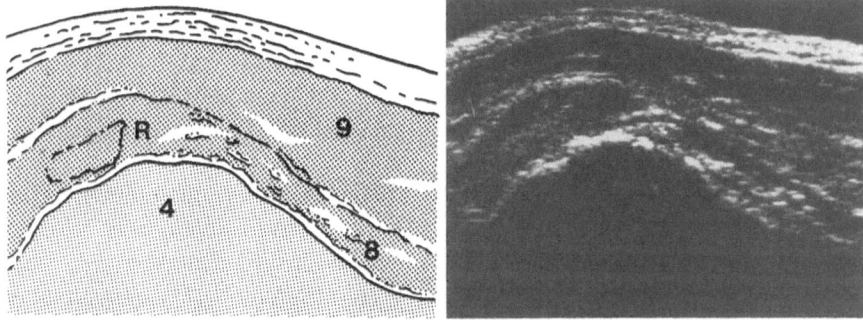

Fig. 39. Fresh rupture of the long biceps tendon. Anterior longitudinal scan. The distal tendon stump shows an irregular echo pattern. The recess of the long biceps tendon (**R**) is filled with anechoic and hypoechoic structures. The irregularly shaped echogenic structure probably represents clotted blood. **4** Proximal humerus, **8** long biceps tendon, **9** deltoid muscle

Dislocations of the Shoulder (Figs. 40, 41; see Figs. 22, 23)

With ultrasound, the bony contour of the proximal humerus and the surrounding soft tissues can be examined immediately after reduction of the shoulder without pain and without special positioning.

Hill-Sachs lesions occur on the posterior or posterolateral aspect of the humeral head and can be visualized without superimposing other structures (see Fig. 22). The dynamic posterior transverse scan will disclose whether the lesion engages against the glenoid surface of the scapula with external rotation of the arm, with a potential for recurrence of the dislocation due to the prying action of the defect.

Avulsion fractures of the greater tuberosity create a stepoff deformity visible on lateral scans. Displacement of the greater tuberosity can block abduction due to impingement of the tuberosity on the acromion (see Fig. 23). Coexisting soft-tissue injuries can be detected early, and subsequent stability testing with comparison of both sides will establish whether the dislocated shoulder can be displaced further from the glenoid.

When operative treatment is proposed, the retroversion of the humeral head should be determined as a prelude to selecting the most appropriate surgical procedure. Pathologically small retroversion angles can predispose to recurrent dislocations, and determination of this angle is important in making a prognosis (Figs. 40 and 41).

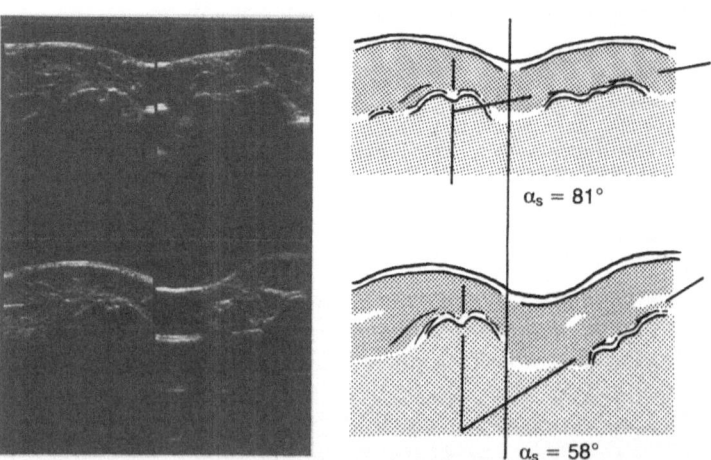

Fig. 40. Sonographic determination of the retroversion angle (α_s) following a Weber rotational osteotomy in the left shoulder. Anterior transverse scan (proximal and distal humerus). The operation was performed for recurrent dislocation of the left shoulder with a large Hill-Sachs lesion. The osteotomy increased the retroversion of the humeral head. The retroversion angle of the left shoulder *(top half of figure)* is increased by 23° relative to the right shoulder. (See also Fig. 41)

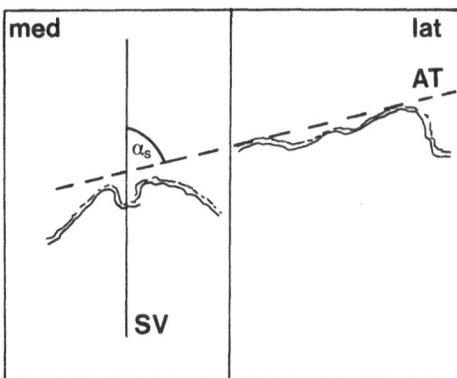

Fig. 41. Determination of the retroversion angle α_s. The anterior contour of the proximal humerus is shown in the *left half of the figure* and the distal humerus in the *right half of the figure*, with medial toward the left. A bubble level is used to maintain the transducer in a horizontal position. The proximal humerus is rotated until the intertubercular sulcus is directed vertically. A line is drawn tangent to the contour of the distal humerus. The retroversion angle α_s is formed by the vertical line through the sulcus (**SV**) and the anterior trochlear tangent (**AT**)

Injuries of the Acromioclavicular Joint (Figs. 42 and 43)

The superior silhouette of the acromioclavicular joint is clearly defined with ultrasound. In a simple contusional injury with no ligamentous tears or displacement, the distended joint capsule forms a prominent arc bridging from the acromion to the clavicle (Fig. 42). When there is ligamentous injury with progressive joint instability, sonography demonstrates elevation of the clavicle with marked incongruity of the bone ends (Figs. 43). The degree of the displacement is easily determined on the scan.

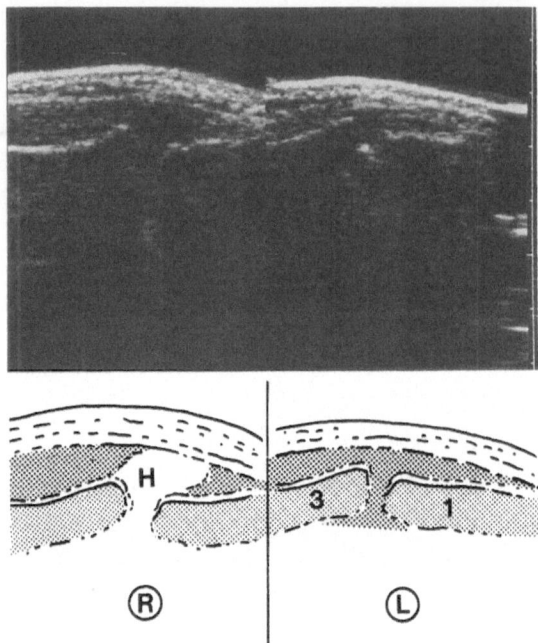

Fig. 42. Contusion of the right acromioclavicular (AC) joint. Scan over the AC joint. After falling from a bicycle onto the right shoulder, the patient experienced tenderness over the right AC joint. There is no incongruity of the AC joint, but a hypoechoic hematoma (H) is visible over the joint space. The uninjured left side is shown for comparison. **1** Acromion, **3** acromial end of clavicle

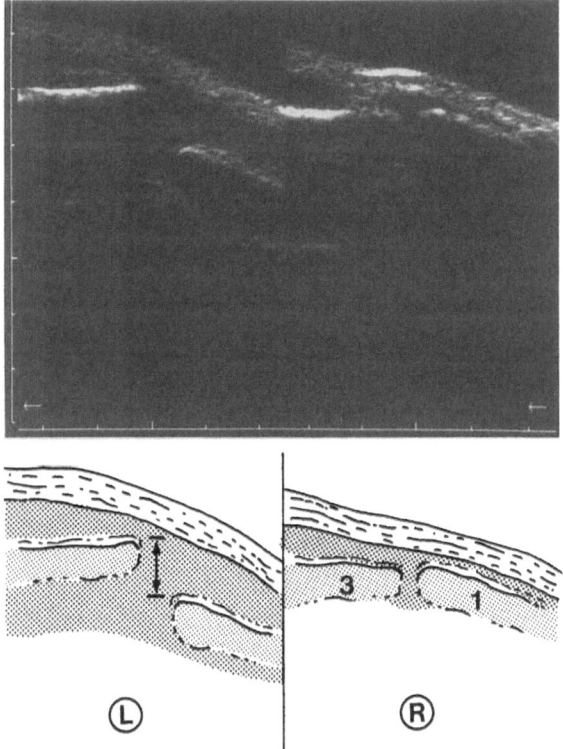

Fig. 43. Dislocation of the AC joint (Tossy grade III). Coronal scan. A prominent step is seen between the AC joint surfaces on the injured left side (**arrow**). The normal right side is shown for comparison. **1** Acromion, **3** acromial end of clavicle

References

Crass JR, CraigEV, Thompson R, Feinberg SB (1984) Ultrasonography of the rotator cuff: surgical correlation. J Clin Ultrasound 12: 487-492

Dähnert W, Bernd W (1986) Computertomographische Bestimmungen des Torsionswinkels am Humerus. Z Orthop 124: 46-49

Morscher E (ed) (1979) Funktionelle Diagnostik in der Orthopädie. Kongreßbericht der 66. Tagung, DGOT Basel 1979, Enke, Stuttgart

Gegenbaur C (1968) Über die Drehung des Humerus. Jenaische Z Med Naturwissenschaft 4: 50-64

Habermayer P, Mayer R, Mayr B, Brunner U, Sachs G (1984) Comparative diagnosis of rotator muscle injuries using arthrography, CT and sonography. Z Unfallchir Versicherungsmed Berufskr 77: 121-129

Harland U (1986) Die sonographische Untersuchung des Schultergelenkes. Med Orthop Techn 2

Hedtmann A, Weber A, Schleberger R (1985) Möglichkeiten der Ultraschalldiagnostik am Schultergelenk. In: Kölbel R (ed) 2. Hamburger Schulterworkshop, Feb. 1985. 3M-Deutschland, Neuss

Hirschfelder H (1986) Erweitertes Spektrum der Schulterdiagnostik mit Hilfe der Computertomographie. Electromedica 54: 90-95

Kramps HA, Laumann U (1983) Morphologische Veränderungen des Gleno-Humeralgelenkes bei habitueller Schulterluxation - Eine computertomographische Studie. Z Orthop 121: 454

Laurence A, Mack MD et al. (1985) US evaluation of the rotator cuff. Radiology 157: 205-209

Middleston WD, Edelstein G, Reinus WR, Melson GL, Murphy WA (1984) Ultrasound of the rotator cuff: technique and normal appearance. J Ultrasound Med 3: 549-551

Weber BG (1971) Humerusosteotomie bei habitueller Schulterluxation. Ther Umsch 28: 292-293

Elbow Joint

Technique of Examination

The elbow joint is evaluated on continuous longitudinal and transverse scans performed over the anterior and posterior aspects of the joint. The following longitudinal scans are standard:

- longitudinal scan over the posterior aspect of the olecranon, olecranon fossa, and humeral shaft;
- longitudinal scan over the radial head, radial fossa, and capitellum from the anterior aspect of the humeroradial joint;
- longitudinal scan over the ulna, coronoid process, trochlea, and coronoid fossa of the humeroulnar joint from the anterior side.

Joint motion studies are essential, and may be accomplised on the posterior longitudinal scan. For this examination the transducer is applied longitudinally over the humeral shaft and olecranon while the examiner's free hand moves the patient's forearm slowly in flexion and extension. During extension the olecranon is seen to glide over the trochlea of the humerus into the olecranon fossa.

The dynamic examination allows a more precise identification of the true joint space. This is most easily done from the posterior aspect; anterior scans are less satisfactory for joint space evaluations. A small contact area between transducer and skin is preferable for dynamic studies.

The brachial artery courses between the brachioradialis and supinator muscles and appearas as a longitudinal tubular structure containing low-level echoes. It is a useful landmark and aid to orientation, and its pulsations provide a "blinking light" in the darkness of the soft tissues.

Interpretive Criteria

Inflammatory changes lead to enhaced sound transmission in the elbow region.
The following sonographic signs may be identified (Figs. 44 and 45):

- thickening of the synovial membrane;
- increased echogenicity of bony surfaces;
- disruption of cortical echoes by a bony lesion that is accessible to the ultrasound beam (the beam is reflected from the base of the defect);
- hypotrophied muscle becomes more echogenic with less sharply defined
  boundaries;
- inflammatory substrate fills and outlines the joint spaces;
- inflammatory substrate fills certain areas in the joint, especially the recesses
  above the trochlea, making the proximal portion of the joint space easier to
  define (Fig. 46).

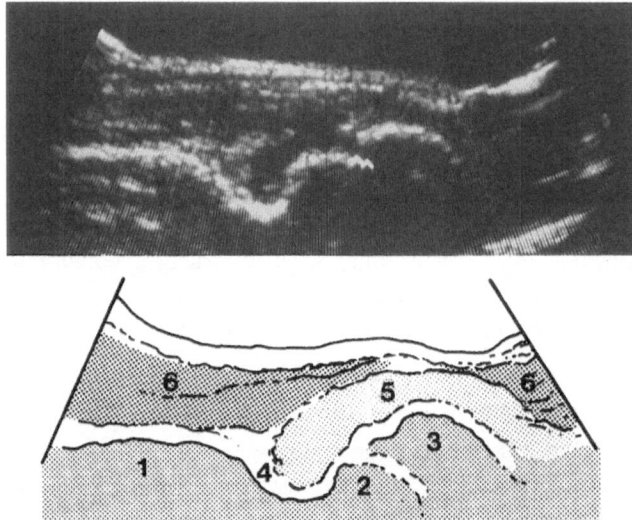

Fig. 44. Elbow involvement in rheumatoid arthritis, posterior longitudinal scan over the
humeral shaft and olecranon with the joint in extension. **1** Humeral shaft, **2** trochlea of
humerus, **3** olecranon, **4** olecranon fossa, **5** inflammatory substrate, **6** muscle

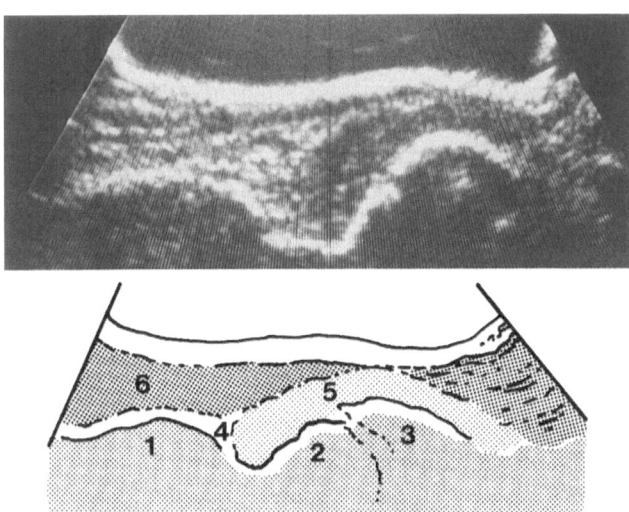

Fig. 45. Elbow involvement in rheumatoid arthritis, posterior longitudinal scan with the joint in flexion. **1** Humeral shaft, **2** trochlea of humerus, **3** olecranon, **4** olecranon fossa, **5** inflammatory substrate, **6** muscle

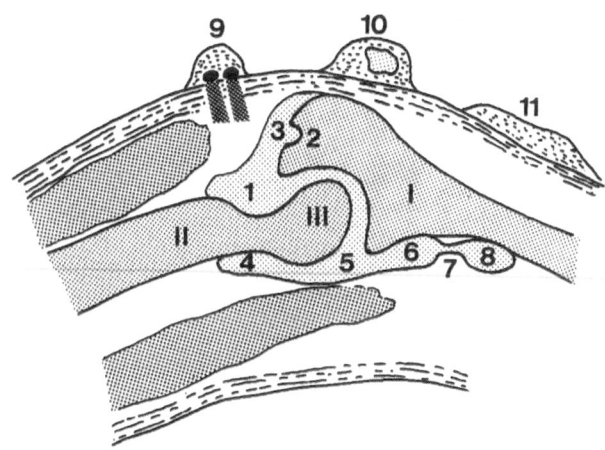

Fig. 46. Summary of pathologic changes that may be detected in the elbow joint. **I** Olecranon, **II** humeral shaft, **III** humeral trochlea, **1** inflammatory substrate in the olecranon fossa, **2** bone defect, **3** synovitis over the olecranon, **4** synovitis in the coronoid fossa, **5** synovitis in the anterior joint space, **6** expanded anterior inferior recess with inflammatory change, **7** channel communicating with cyst, **8** cubital synovial cyst, **9** gouty tophus with typical acoustic shadow, **10** olecranon bursitis: combination of anechoic, hypoechoic, and highly echogenic internal structures producing a very nonhomogeneous, irregular echo pattern, **11** rheumatic nodule: homogeneous, tubular structure of low echogenicity

Normal Sonographic Anatomy

Although the elbow joint consists of three separate articulations, its anatomy is plainly defined on posterior and anterior transverse scans. The following standard scans are additionally recommended:

Posterior Longitudinal Scan

This scan demonstrates:
- the humeral shaft as an echogenic structure with a distal acoustic shadow;
- the olecranon fossa as a small, echogenic hollow extending to the end of the humeral shaft;
- the olecranon as an echogenic structure at the proximal end of the ulna with a hook-shaped superior border;
- the triceps muscle as a hypoechoic structure with the typical echotexture of muscle tissue;
- the trochlea as a circular bony structure with an acoustic shadow, which blends partly or completely with the olecranon shadow depending on the joint position;
- the joint space as a faint, hypoechoic band between the trochlea and olecranon;
- the proximal hyaline cartilage as a weakly echogenic band no more than 2 mm thick covering the articular surface of the trochlea (Fig. 47).

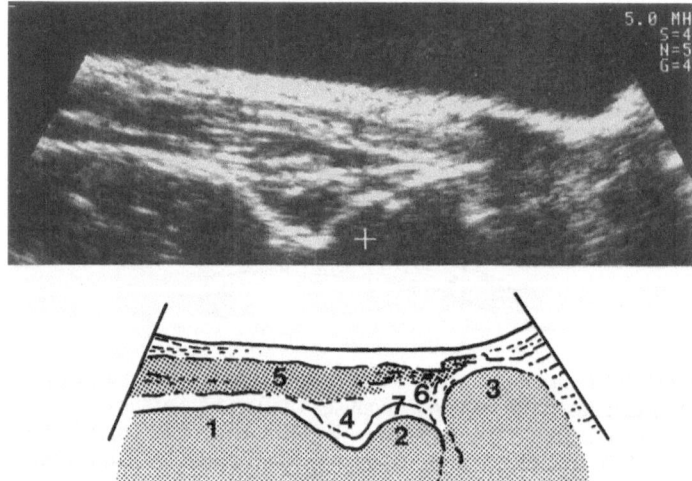

Fig. 47. Normal humeroulnar joint, posterior scan. **1** Humeral shaft, **2** humeral trochlea, **3** olecranon, **4** olecranon fossa, **5** triceps muscle, **6** joint space, **7** peritrochlear hyaline cartilage

Anterior Longitudinal Scan

This scan, performed over the humeroradial joint and then over the humeroul-nar joint, demonstrates:
- the trochlea as an echogenic arc with adjacent shadowing;
- the humeral shaft as a straight line of bright echoes with adjacent shadow-ing;
- the coronoid fossa between the humeral shaft and trochlea;
- the ulna as a line of bright echoes distal to the joint with distal shadowing;
- the radial head as a small, round, hooklike feature with distal shadowing;
- the radial fossa between the humeral shaft and trochlea, known also as the capitellum in the area of the humeroradial joint;
- the anterior muscles of the elbow joint, consisting of the biceps, brachialis, and brachioradialis, which are poorly distinguishable from one another on sonograms (Figs. 48 and 49).

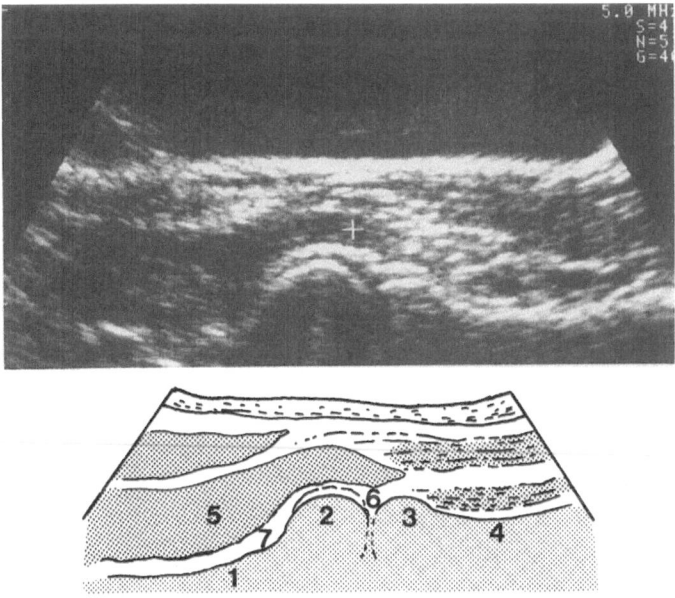

Fig. 48. Normal humeroradial joint, anterior scan. **1** Humeral shaft, **2** capitellum, **3** ra-dial head, **4** radial shaft, **5** muscle, **6** joint space, **7** radial fossa

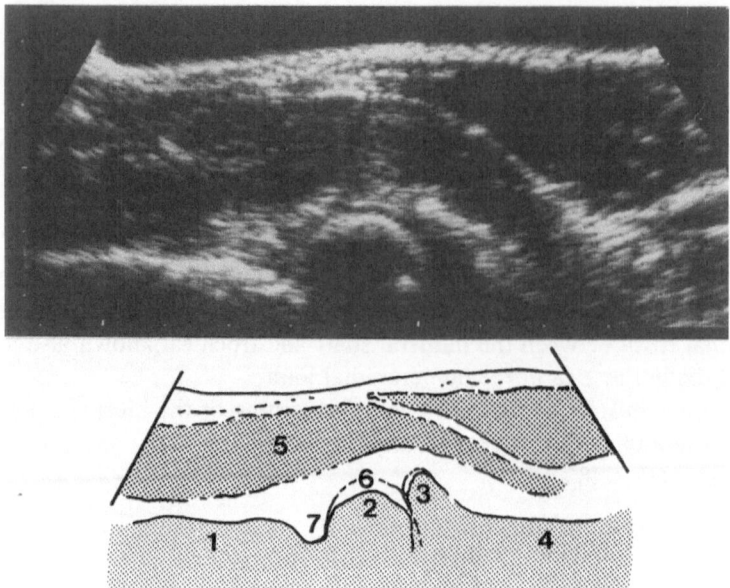

Fig. 49. Normal humeroulnar joint, anterior scan. **1** Humeral shaft, **2** humeral trochlea, **3** ulnar coronoid process, **4** ulnar shaft, **5** muscle, **6** peritrochlear hyaline cartilage, **7** coronoid fossa

Pathologic Conditions

Cubital Arthritis

Inflammatory changes in the humeroulnar and humeroradial joints can be diagnosed by noting the sonographic signs of inflammation. These are best appreciated on the posterior longitudinal scan over the olecranon fossa, which in the presence of inflammation appears hypoechoic or echo-free. Areas involved by synovitis appear less echogenic than the adjacent triceps muscle tissue (Figs. 50–52).

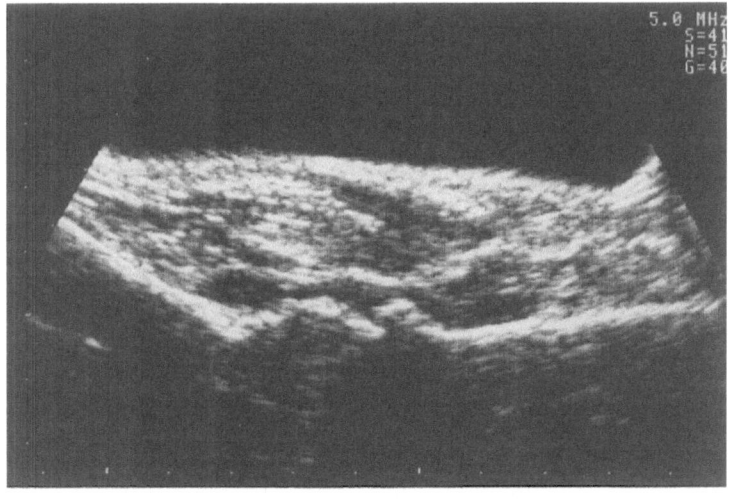

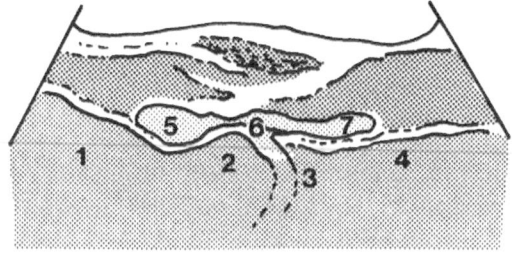

Fig. 50. Arthritis of the humeroulnar joint, anterior longitudinal scan. **1** Humeral shaft, **2** humeral trochlea, **3** proximal ulna with coronoid process, **4** ulnar shaft, **5** inflammatory substrate in coronoid fossa, **6** joint space, **7** expanded inferior recess

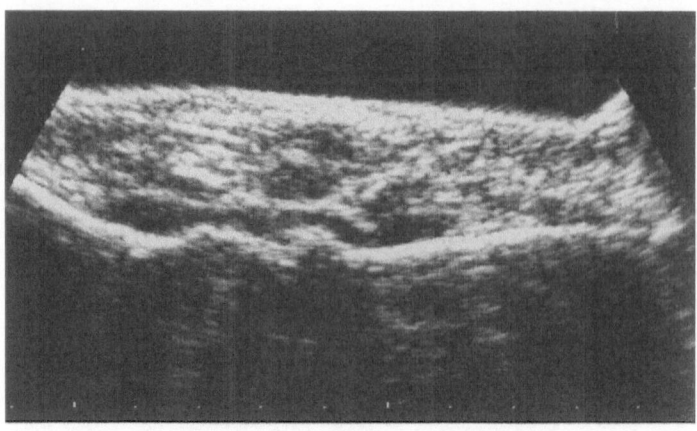

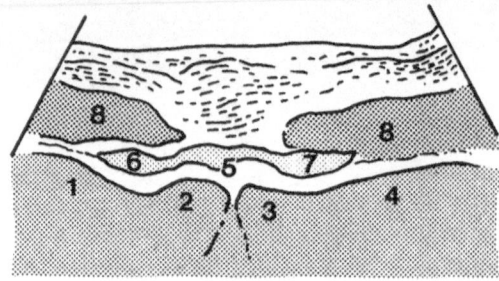

Fig. 51. Cubital arthritis, anterior longitudinal scan of humeroradial joint in seropositive rheumatoid arthritis. **1** Humeral shaft, **2** capitellum, **3** radial head, **4** radial shaft, **5** inflammatory substrate over joint space, **6** inflammatory substrate in radial fossa, **7** expanded inferior recess, **8** muscle

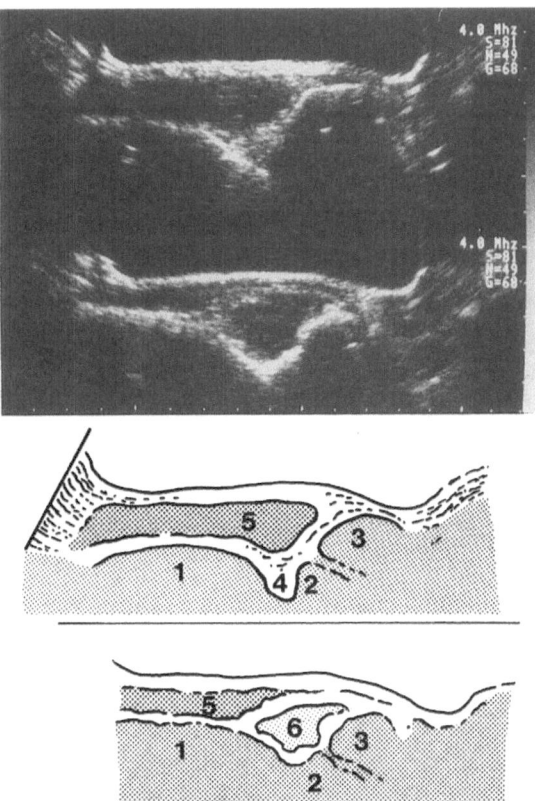

Fig. 52. Comparison of normal findings *(top)* with cubital arthritis *(bottom)* in a 59-year-old woman with seropositive rheumatoid arthritis. There is inflammatory substrate (6) in the olecranon fossa. **1** Humeral shaft, **2** humeral trochlea, **3** olecranon, **4** olecranon fossa, **5** triceps muscle

Destructive Lesions in Arthritis

Bone destruction in arthritis is characterized by irregular deformity with defects and erosive changes in the olecranon and the intrusion of inflammatory material into the bone defects. The destructive effect of synovitis, called pannus, can be directly visualized with ultrasound (Fig. 53).

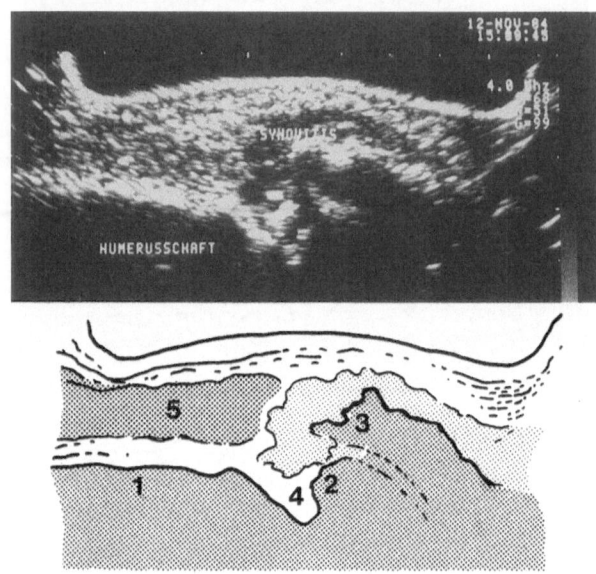

Fig. 53. Seventy-seven year old woman with seropositive rheumatoid arthritis, stage IV, destructive cubital arthritis, posterior longitudinal scan, elbow in extension. **1** Humeral shaft, **2** trochlea, **3** remnant of olecranon, **4** olecranon fossa, **5** muscle. *Humerusschaft:* Humeral shaft

Cyst Formation

Continuous anterior longitudinal scans also provide direct visualization of inflammatory changes in the humeroradial and humeroulnar joints. It is common in such cases to find a cystic lesion anterior to the radius below the radial head. Most of the lesions communicate with the joint space, but a few are entirely separate from it. These are synovial cysts, easily identifiable by percutaneous aspiration and cytologic analysis. It is believed that cysts of the elbow region form in many cases where cubital arthritis is advanced and of long duration. The cysts, whether they communicate with the joint space or are separate from it, may result from a gravitational effect on the inflammatory material (Fig. 54).

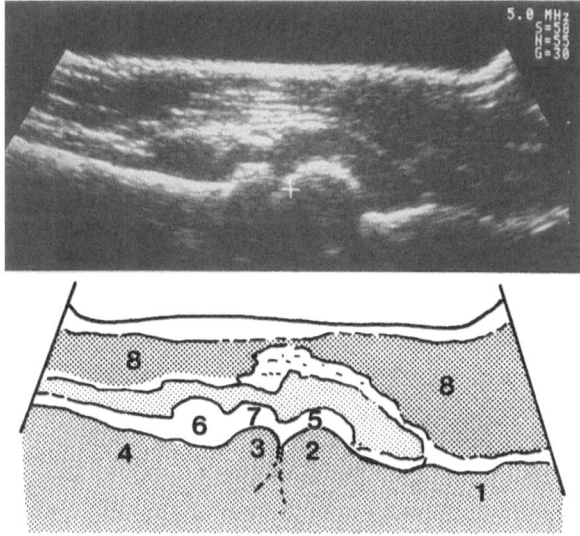

Fig. 54. Sixty-eight year old woman with seropositive rheumatoid arthritis and cubital synovial cyst formation over the radial shaft, anterior longitudinal scan. **1** Humeral shaft, **2** capitellum, **3** radial head, **4** radial shaft, **5** inflammatory substrate, **6** cubital synovial cyst, **7** connecting channel, **8** muscle

Bursitis

In some cases an irregular, hypoechoic mass is found posterior to the olecra-non. This structure transmits sound well to the surface of the underlying bone and is strictly localized to this region. Its internal echo pattern is usually hetero-geneous. Very hypoechoic to anechoic areas in the mass alternate with hyper-echoic areas (Fig. 55).

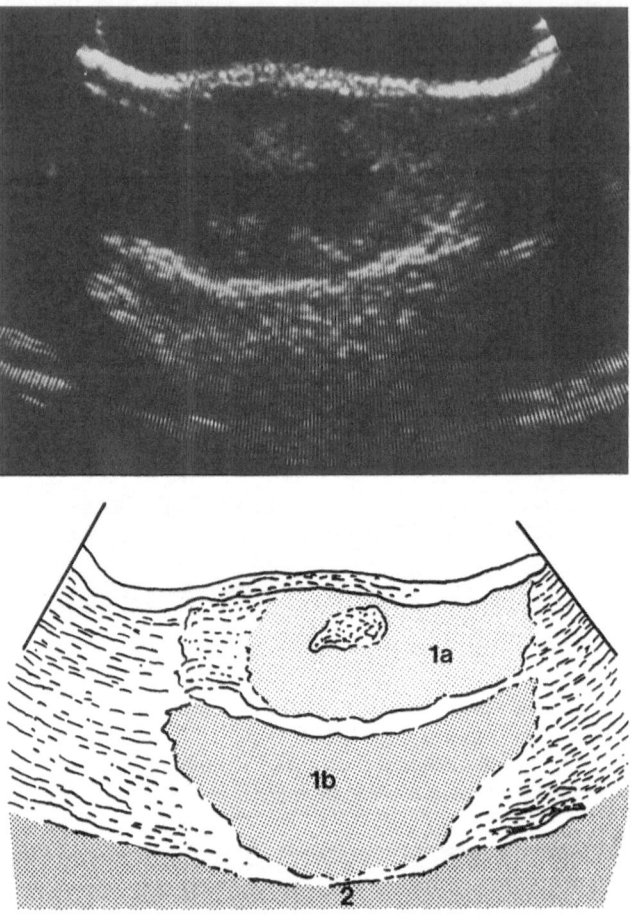

Fig. 55. Olecranon bursitis. The echo pattern is heteregeneous, with consists of echo-free areas (**1a**, fluid) alternating with more echogenic structures (**1b**, cellular substrate and fi-brin). **1** Olecranon bursitis, **2** olecranon

Rheumatic Nodules

These lesions occur mostly on the posterior border of the proximal ulna. They are homogeneous, typically round to oval in shape but sometimes tubular, and always hypoechoic. They move little when palpated (Fig. 56).

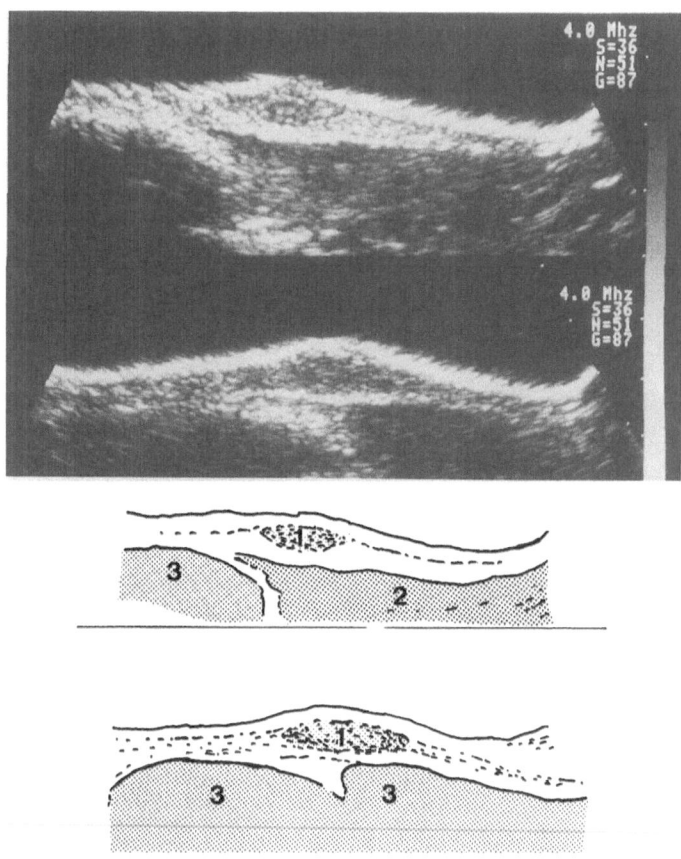

Fig. 56. Bilateral rheumatic nodule formation at a typical site, the posterior ulnar border. **1** Rheumatic nodule, **2** muscle, **3** bone

Gouty Tophus

This lesion appears as a hyperechoic nodule with distal acoustic shadowing (Table 3, Fig. 57).

Table 3. Arthrosonographic differentiation of rheumatic nodules, bursitis, and gouty tophi

Diagnosis	Sonographic features
Rheumatic nodules	Sharply marginated, homogeneous structures of low echogenicity
Bursitis	Irregularly shaped area with heterogeneous echo pattern. Margins are usually indistinct. Anechoic to hypoechoic areas alternate with sonodense areas
Gouty tophi	Hyperechoic nodules with acoustic shadowing of variable intensity

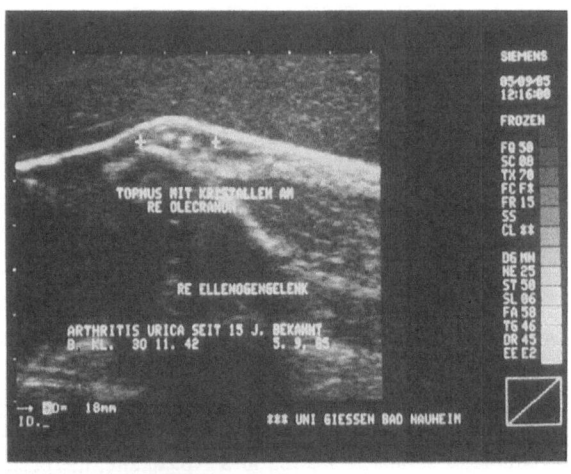

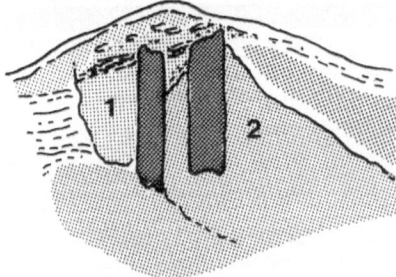

Fig. 57. Gouty tophus on the elbow, hyperechoic nodule casting partial shadows on the olecranon. **1** Gouty tophus, **2** olecranon

Comments

The various inflammatory rheumatic disorders that involve the elbow joint cannot be positively differentiated by arthrosonography, and the evaluation of all available findings is necessary for an accurate differential diagnosis (Fig. 58).

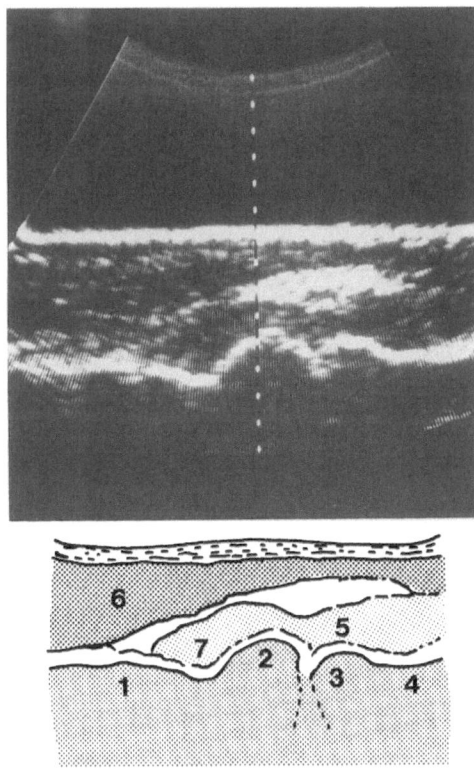

Fig. 58. Severe cubital arthritis in rheumatoid arthritis, anterior longitudinal scan. **1** Humeral shaft, **2** capitellum, **3** radial head, **4** radial shaft, **5** inflammatory substrate, **6** muscle, **7** radial fossa

References

Pirani M, Lange-Meckler I, Cockshott WP (1982) Rupture of a posterior synovial cyst of the elbow. J Rheumatol 9/1: 94–96

Sattler H, Spielmann G (1985a) Zur Wertigkeit der Sonographie in der Differenzierung nodulärer Veränderungen bei entzündlich rheumatischen Erkrankungen. Ultraschalldiagnostik 85. Thieme, Stuttgart, p 636

Sattler H, Spielmann G (1985b) Die Arthrosonographie des Ellbogengelenkes – Grenzen und Möglichkeiten. Ultraschalldiagnostik 85. Thieme, Stuttgart p 652

Sattler H, Schmidt KL (1986) Status of arthrosonography in rheumatologic diagnosis: examination technic, findings and their interpretation. I. The elbow joint. Zum Stellenwert der Arthrosonographie in der rheumatologischen Diagnostik: Untersuchungstechnik, Befunde und ihre Interpretation. I. Ellbogengelenk. Z Rheumatol 45 (1): 1–6

Seltzer SE, Finberg HJ, Weissmann BN (1980) Arthrosonography – technique, sonographic anatomy and pathology. Invest Radiol 15: 19–28

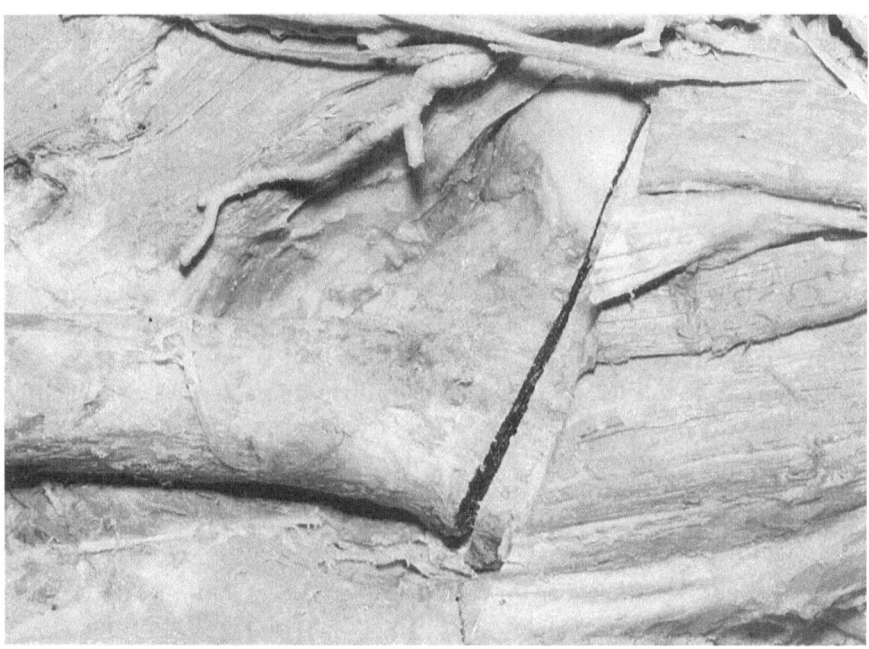

Fig. 59. Anatomic specimen of a left hip. The hip flexor muscles have been dissected free. The saw cut follows the approximate plane of the ultrasound scan

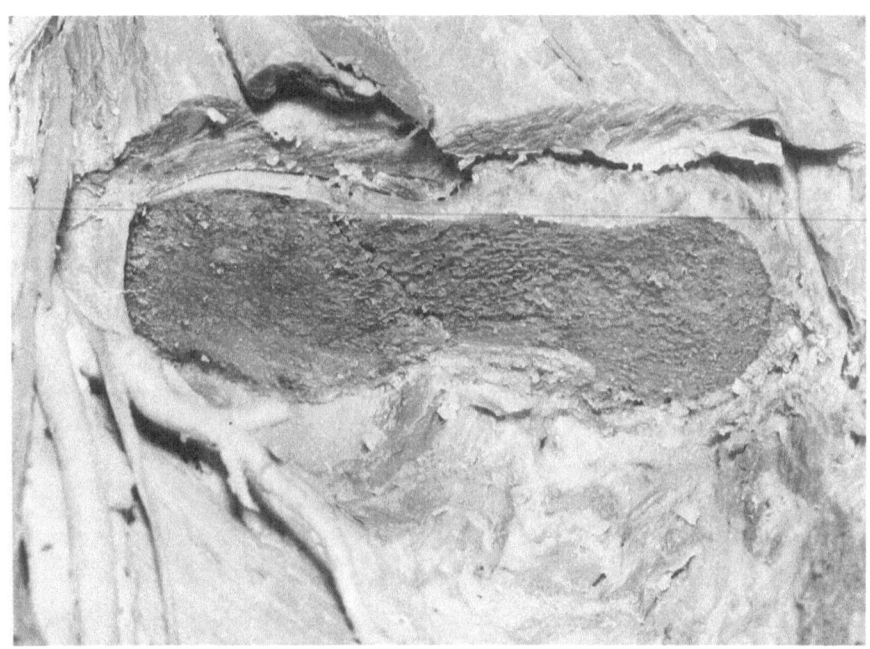

Hip Joint in Children, Adolescents, and Adults

Technique of Examination

The examination is performed with a 5-MHz transducer. A standoff pad is not essential since the structures of interest lie 2–4 cm below the skin surface and thus within the focal zone of the probe.

The hip can be imaged on numerous planes of section. Because the acetabulum is directed anteriorly and gives scant bony coverage to the anterior part of the femoral head, and because of the physiologic anteversion of the femoral neck, anterior sonograms can define a large portion of the femoral head. For anatomic reasons, then, it is recommended that the hip be scanned from the anterior aspect (Figs. 59 and 60).

The transducer is applied so that its medial end is over the approximate center of the inguinal ligament and its long axis is parallel to the axis of the femoral neck (Fig. 61). On this plane the femoral head appears as a semicircular feature in the medial part of the scan and is continuous laterally with the femoral neck. External rotation of the hip brings the femoral head farther out of the acetabulum, increasing the proportion of the head that is visible with ultrasound. Internal rotation at the hip places the femoral neck on a more horizontal plane, tenses the posterior capsule, and relaxes the anterior capsule. This facilitates the detection of joint effusions.

The femoral anteversion angle can be determined by imaging the femoral neck on a scan parallel to the neck axis. The desired plane is obtained by scanning the femoral neck from below upward in a sweeping fashion until a sharp cortex echo is defined. Anteversion is determined in the supine position with the knees flexed 90° over the edge of the table. The transducer is positioned horizontally with the aid of a bubble level, and the angle of inclination of the femoral neck is measured. If the anteversion angle is large, the transducer should be positioned parallel to the femoral neck and the inclination of the neck relative to the horizontal (the anteversion angle as defined by Rönig) determined with a goniometric level (Fig. 61). Otherwise the femoral neck will form too great an angle with the incident sound waves, and a sharply defined echo will not be obtained.

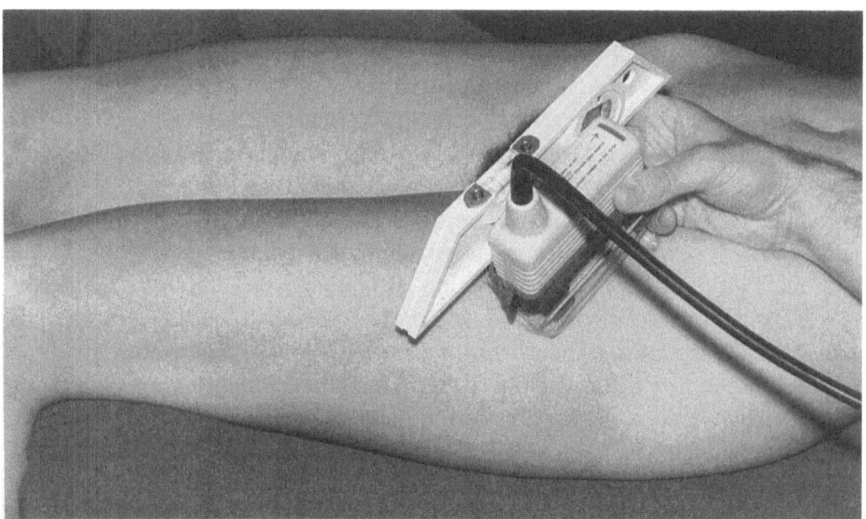

Fig. 61. The transducer is positioned parallel to the femoral neck. This scan gives a good view of the joint capsule and the anterior portions of the proximal femur. The same placement is used to determine the anteversion of the femoral neck. For this the hip is placed in neutral rotation and the knees are flexed 90° with the lower legs parallel. The transducer is either positioned horizontally using a bubble level and the inclination of the femoral neck from the horizontal is measured, or (for large AV angles) it is positioned parallel to the femoral neck, and the inclination of the transducer from the horizontal is measured with a goniometric level

◄———————————————————————————————————

Fig. 60. Same specimen as in Fig. 59 with the distal femur removed. Viewed from below, the cut surface shows the structures visualized on a scan plane following the axis of the femoral neck. The tensor fasciae latae overlies the bone surface laterally, and the iliopsoas medially. The sartorius and rectus femoris intervene superficially between the tensor fasciae latae and iliopsoas

Normal Sonographic Anatomy

The critical landmarks for sonographic evaluations of the hip are the femoral head, which appears semicircular, and the femoral neck, which adjoins the femoral head laterally and forms almost a straight line (Figs. 60 and 62).

In infants the femoral head of very low echogenicity. With appearance of the capital femoral ossification center, the echo-poor rim of cartilage around the ossification center becomes progressively narrowed, as does the epiphyseal plate, until the end of the growth period. By puberty the epiphyseal plate divides the semicircular femoral head approximately in half, and the epiphysis is surrounded by about a 1-2 mm rim of cartilage. Sound waves normal to the surface of the femoral head yield a strong echo, while adjacent waves yield less intense echoes. Hence the portion of the head nearest the transducer appears bright, the echogenicity falling off with distance from that point. The head is adjoined laterally by the femoral neck, appearing as a line of bright echoes. The femoral neck should appear as straight as possible, i.e., the scan should cut the femoral neck on a plane that closely aligns with the longitudinal neck axis.

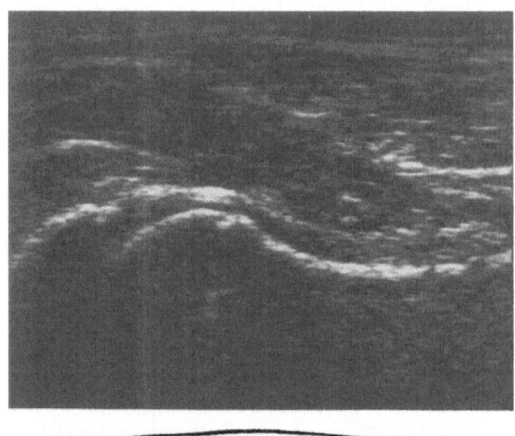

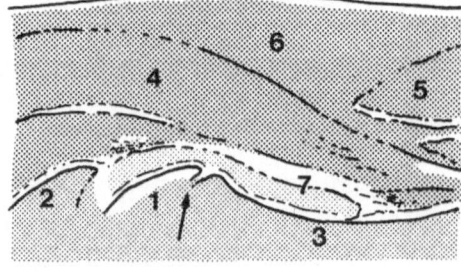

Fig. 62. Normal sonographic findings in a 12-year-old girl. The anterior scan follows the axis of the femoral neck (see Fig. 60). The epiphyseal plate is still open (**arrow**). 1 Epiphysis, 2 ilium, 3 femoral neck, 4 iliopsoas muscle, 5 tensor fasciae latae, 6 sartorius and rectus femoris, 7 joint capsule

At a higher level the intertrochanteric line is demonstrated as a protrusion of varying prominence on the femoral neck in the area of attachment of the joint capsule. On still higher secitons the femoral neck assumes a curved shape and is bounded medially by the femoral head and laterally by the greater trochanter.

Medial to the femoral head is the anterior rim of the acetabulum, represented by a bright cortical echo with shadowing of deeper structures. In children the bony part of the acetabulum is surmounted by a cone-shaped echofree border representing the hyaline cartilage.

The joint capsule closely overlies the bony structures. It appears as an echogenic band that is relatively wide at the acetabulum, narrows greatly over the center of the femoral head, and widens to about 1 mm over the femoral neck. The synovium of the hip joint appears as a hypoechoic strip about 5 mm wide between the bony structures and the capsule.

Superficial to the capsule are the three large muscle groups of the iliopsoas, the tensor fascia lata, and the saratorius with the rectus femoris.

The iliopsoas forms a band that is wide medially and tapers to a point in its lateral course over the head and neck of the femur.

The muscular septa are hyperechoic, their echoes appearing elongated owing to the oblique incidence of the ultrasound beam relative to the direction of the fibers.

The tensor fascia latae appears as a laterally based triangle which overlies the iliopsoas and whose apex extends medially as far as the femoral head. The sartorius and rectus femoris form a superficial layer at the center of the image, appearing as a narrow band that widens at the center or as an anteriorly based equilateral triangle. The muscular septa are hyperechoic, their echoes appearing as points because the scan is transaxial to the direction of the muscle fibers.

Real-time scans may show the pulsation of the ascending branch of the lateral circumflex femoral artery lateral to the femoral head between the capsule and the iliopsoas muscle.

Interpretive Criteria

It has proved helpful to evaluate scans in terms of the following types of finding:

- soft-tissue changes
- changes in the joint cavity,
- osseous changes,
- epiphyseal growth disturbances, and
- measurement of anteversion.

Soft-tissue changes can often be detected on the standard anterior view. This plane is optimum for defining the relationship of cystic lesions to the joint capsule. The relationship of abscesses or cysts to the femoral artery is best appreciated on other planes (e.g., a scan over the longitudinal course of the femoral artery).

Disorders that are associated with enlargement of the *joint cavity* are seen to good advantage on the anterior scan (Figs. 63 and 64). The parallel course of the femoral neck and joint capsule makes it easy to recognize a change in the distance between them, the normal distance being approximately 5 mm. Values of 10 mm or more are definitely pathologic. The portion of the capsule lateral to the femoral head can undergo greater expansion than the medial portion due to the restraining action of the iliofemoral ligament. Besides the volume of the effusion, the degree of lateral capsular expansion depends on the joint posi-

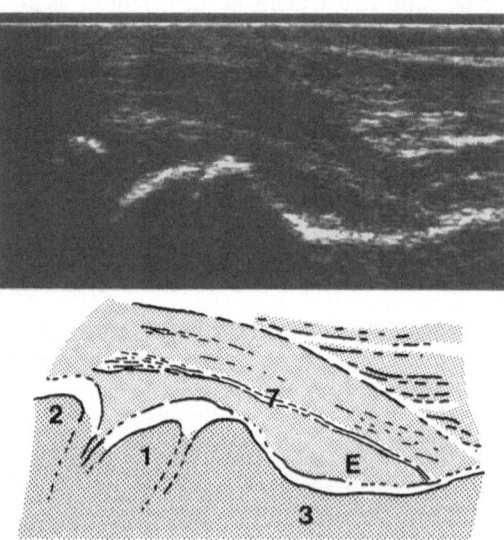

Fig. 63. Coxitis fugax, anterior scan on the femoral neck axis. The 5-year-old boy developed a painful hip 2 weeks after an influenzal infection. Aspirate from the joint was sterile. Ultrasound shows distension of the joint capsule (7) by an effusion (E). **1** Epiphysis, **2** ilium, **3** femoral neck

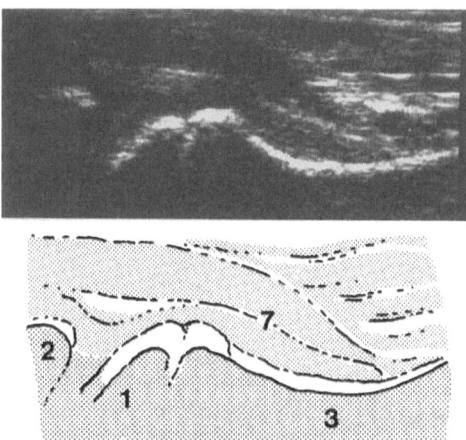

Fig. 64. Same patient as in Fig. 63, 1 week later. Anterior scan on the femoral neck axis. The distance between the femoral neck (3) and hip joint capsule (7) has diminished, and the intracapsular space appears more echogenic than in Fig. 63. By this time the patient was asymptomatic. **1** Epipyhsis, **2** ilium

tion. External rotation tenses the anterior parts of the capsule and relaxes the posterior parts, while internal rotation has the opposite effects.

Osseous changes such as osteophytes and cortical defects are appreciated only if they occur in the anterior sector encompassed by the scan (see Figs. 65 and 66). The sector covers an angle of approximately 60°.

Cortical defects in the femoral head like those occurring in the fragmentation stage of Perthes' disease or in avascular necrosis of the femoral head in adults create a discontinuity in the smooth echogenic contour of the bone. Earlier stages of diminished blood flow to the femoral head and cancellous bone remodeling are not visualized. It is unclear how often such changes are associated with irritation of the joint and sonographically detectable expansion of the capsule.

Cortical defects in the femoral head have the same shape and appearance as in other joints. The majority are rounded with sharply defined margins.

Osteophytes likewise disrupt the smooth cortical surface, creating an irregularity that is convex rather than concave as in the case of bone defects.

Epiphyseal growth disturbances occur in enchondral dysostoses, Perthes' disease, and slipping of the capital femoral epiphysis. They produce typical sonographic changes in the femoral head and neck. During the period from the appearance of the capital femoral ossification center to closure of the epiphyseal plate, the ratio of bony metaphysis to ossified epiphysis changes, attaining a value of approximately 1:1 at skeletal maturity. Lateral disparities in this ratio may provide early sonographic evidence of Perthes' disease. The ratio of epiphysis to metaphysis is also changed in enchondral dysostoses. In this case the disturbance is symmetrical, however, and diagnosis must rely on a comparison with children of approximately equal age.

Slipping of the capital femoral epiphysis creates a step at the level of the epiphysis, the height of the step being proportional to the degree of slip (see Fig. 70). If the hip is being scanned on the plane of the slip, a step of 1 mm correspondes to a slip of approximately 5°.

The positioning technique for the *measurement of femoral anteversion* is described under Technique of Examination on p. 65.

Pathologic Conditions

Hip Dysplasia

The infant hip can be evaluated sonographically for acetabular development and femoral head coverage using the criteria introduced by Graf. This evaluation cannot be performed in older patients. Femoral anteversion can be determined to identify deviations from the normal range. If the anteversion angle is increased, this finding should be checked radiographically. Osteoarthritis of the hip secondary to dysplasia can lead to joint effusions which will resolve as the arthrotic irritation subsides. The intra-articular fluid collection is manifested by distension of the capsule. Osteophytes occurring in the anterior part of the joint lead to "step formation" in the cortical surface.

Osteoarthritis of the Hip

Osteoarthritis of the hip is characterized by narrowing of the joint space, sclerosis of subchondral structures, osteophyte formation, and cystic changes. Osteophytes and cysts can be visualized with ultrasound only if they cause destruction of femoral head cortex within the sector covered by the anterior scan. Osteophytic changes in the acetabulum tend to affect its superior portion and generally are not displayed on the anterior scan. Osteophytic outgrowths at the junction of the femoral head and neck create a *step* in the normally smooth contour of the proximal femur (Fig. 65). Hip joint effusions may also occur in the setting of osteoarthritis.

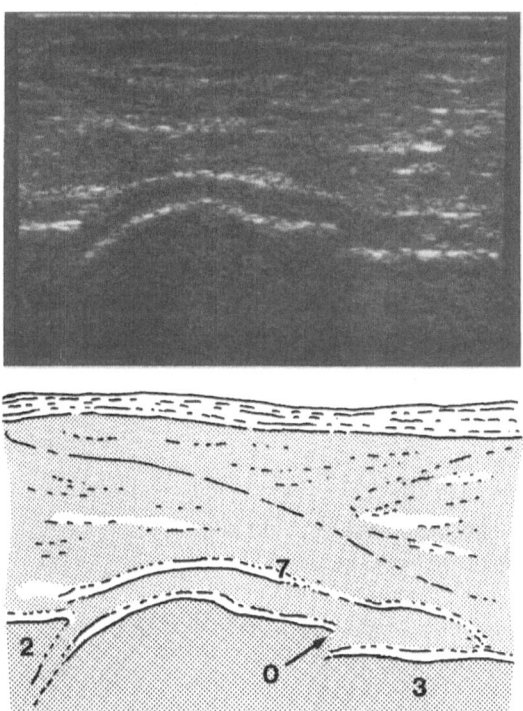

Fig. 65. Osteoarthritis of the hip, anterior scan on the femoral neck axis. An osteophyte (O) has created a steplike discontinuity at the junction of the femoral head and neck. 2 Ilium, 3 femoral neck, 7 joint capsule

Avascular Necrosis of the Femoral Head

Early stages of avascular necrosis in adults are not detectable with ultrasound. In more advanced stages where degenerative joint changes supervene, the sonographic features are like those in osteoarthritis of the hip.

Coxitis

Coxitis may be secondary to rheumatoid disease or infection. The predominant ultrasound finding is joint effusion causing separation of the capsule from the femoral neck. Intracapsular volume changes may be seen in association with:

- rheumatoid arthritis,
- Bekhterev's disease,
- psoriatic arthritis,
- bacterial arthritis,
- reactive arthritis (postinfectious arthritis),
- avasular necrosis of the femoral head,
- hip dysplasias,
- idiopathic osteoarthritis of the hip,
- slipped capital femoral epiphysis, and
- Perthes' disease.

The volume increase itself is not helpful in differentiating among these conditions. Differential diagnosis is aided by additional sonographic changes in the proximal femur such as bone defects, osteophytes, altered epiphyseal-metaphyseal ratio, step formation, and other cortical discontinuities. However, the final diagnosis must rely on the patient's history and the sum of clinical, laboratory, and imaging findings.

Generally the intracapsular fluid collection will appear hypoechoic.

Reactive arthritis may be associated with pronounced separation of the capsule from the femoral neck, which diminishes as symptoms regress (see Figs. 63 and 64). Aspiration of the joint generally does not restore the capsule to a normal position, suggesting that the separation is maintained by a cellular proliferation of the synovium. As long as the distance between the cortex and fibrous capsule is less than 10 mm (measured at the head–neck junction), there is little chance of obtaining sufficient material for laboratory analysis and culture.

The effusions associated with *infectious arthritis* are often more pronounced than in the reactive arthritides and rheumatoid disorders. The capsule is often difficult to define, and occasionally the effusion escapes into the surrounding soft tissues. Necrotic tissues appear as more echogenic structures within the effusion.

Involvement of the hip joint in rheumatoid arthritis usually occurs in cases where the diagnosis is already known (Fig. 66).

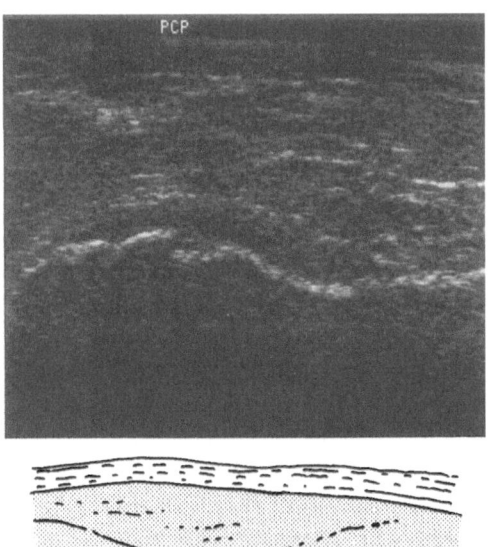

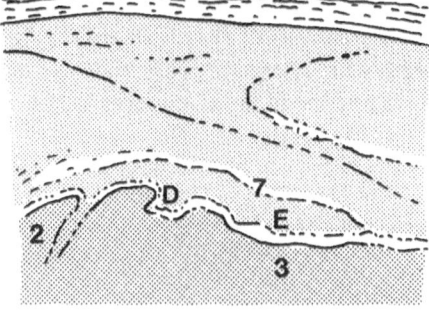

Fig. 66. Hip involvement in rheumatoid arthritis. Anterior scan on the femoral neck axis. The hip joint capsule (**7**) is raised from the femoral neck (**3**) by an intracapsular fluid collection (**E**). The semicircular contour of the femoral head is interrupted by a defect (**D**). **2** Ilium. *PCP:* RA

Hip complaints can occur in the very early stages of *Bekhterev's disease*. When they are associated with marked sonographic elevation of the capsule and minimal radiographic changes, further diagnostic studies should be performed to exclude an ankylosing spondylarthritis.

Epiphyseal Growth Disturbances

These disturbances include *enchondral dysostoses, Perthes' disease,* and *slipped capital femoral epiphysis.*

Enchondral dysostoses are characterized by a general reduction of epiphyseal growth. In the hip joint this is manifested by a flattening of the epiphysis on the anterior scan plane previously described. In Ribbing's disease the cortex of the femoral epiphysis remains intact but is markedly flattened relative to the normal condition. In Fairbank's disease the changes in the epiphysis and metaphysis are similar to those occurring in the fragmentation stage of Perthes' disease.

The sonographic features of the femoral head and neck undergo characteristic changes during the course of *Perthes' disease* (Figs. 67 and 69). In the initial stage the cortex retains its smooth contour. The ratio of epiphysis to metaphysis on the affected side changes in favor of the metaphysis. This occurs because the growth of the ossified epiphysis on the affected side lags behind that on the healthy side. Comparison with the healthy side is always necessary because the ratio of ossified epiphysis to metaphysis changes as growth progresses, and there are no solid data relating these changes to age. (Of course, the examiner

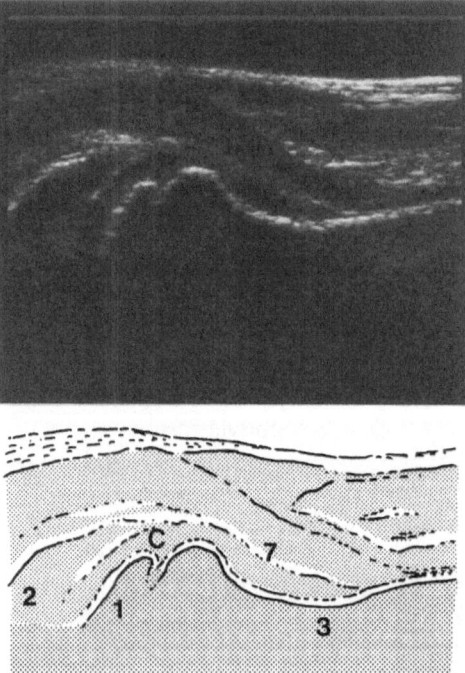

Fig. 67. Perthes' disease, sclerotic stage. Anterior scan on the femoral neck axis. The ossified epiphysis (1) is very flat, the joint capsule (7) undistended. The cartilaginous part of the femoral head (C) is well defined. **2** Ilium, **3** femoral neck

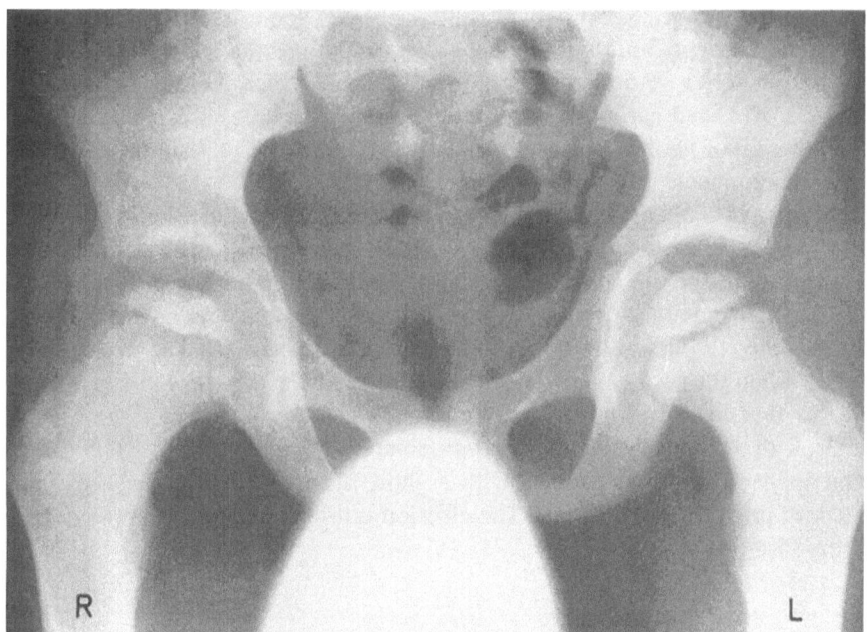

Fig. 68. Roentgenogram of the patient in Fig. 67

should remain alert to the possibility of bilateral disease.) The epiphyseal cortex remains intact in the early stages of Perthes' disease, presenting sonographically as a smooth line of bright echoes. In the fragmentation stage the epiphyseal ossification center is necrotic, and zones of sonolucency appear (Fig. 69).

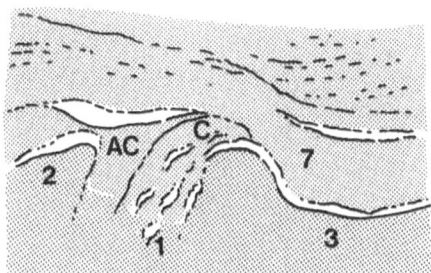 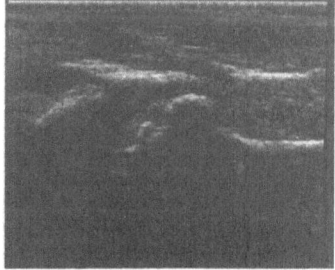

Fig. 69. Perthes' disease, fragmentation stage. Anterior scan on the femoral neck axis. The normally smooth cortical boundary of the epiphysis (**1**) is disrupted, and the epiphysis shows a mottled pattern of echogenicity. The echo-free hyaline cartilage (**C**) is well delineated with respect to the hypoechoic epiphysis and the cartilaginous growth plate of the acetabular roof (**AC**). **2** Ilium, **3** femoral neck, **7** joint capsule

The epiphyseal nucleus is no longer uniformly echogenic, but shows an alternation between hypo- and hyperechoic areas. In 2 of the 11 cases of Perthes' disease in our series we observed a hip joint effusion, which presented the typical features described earlier. It remains unclear whether the effusion constitutes an early sign of Perthes' disease. In later stages it appears to result from insufficient containment.

In over 90% of cases of *slipped capital femoral epiphysis* the femoral neck is displaced superiorly and anteriorly relative to the epiphysis. The normal sonogram in adolscents is characterized by a semicircular contour of the femoral head, which contains a central epiphyseal plate. Displacement of the epiphysis causes a step to form at the level of the plate (Figs. 70 and 71). The step appears largest when the scan is performed on the plane of the slip. In this case the degree of the slip corresponds to the radiographically established displacement angle, with a 1-mm step signifying approximately 5° of slip. We found concomitant joint effusions in patients with a short history (slip occuring less than 1 month prior to examination). The effusion did not correlate with the degree of the slip.

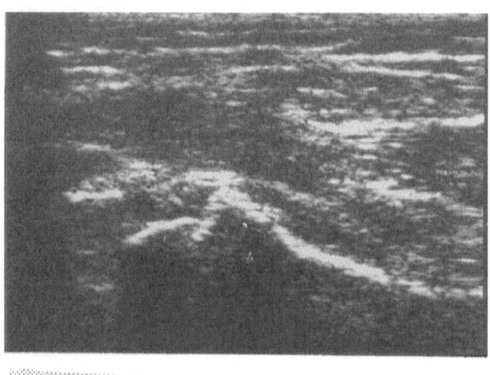

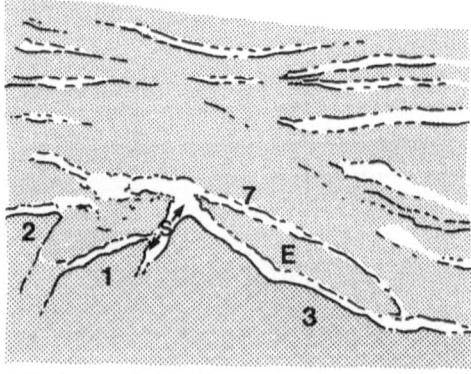

Fig. 70. Slipped capital femoral epiphysis. Anterior scan on the femoral neck axis. The epiphysis (1) is displaced by the distance s relative to the rest of the femoral neck (3) and head. The joint capsule (7) is raised from the femoral neck by an intracapsular fluid collection (E). 2 Ilium

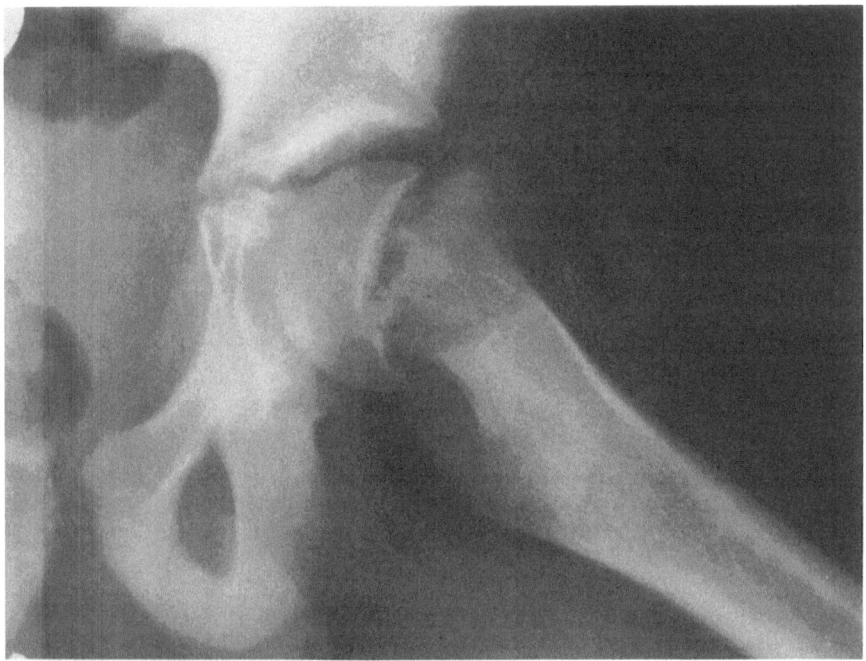

Fig. 71. Roentgenogram of the patient in Fig. 70

References

Endler F et al. (1984) Vermessung von Hüftröntgenbildern. Orthop Röntgendiagnostik 5: 16-5.29

Graf R (1983) Die sonographische Beurteilung der Hüftdysplasie mit Hilfe der "Erker-diagnostik". Z Orthop 121: 693-702

König G, Schult W (1973) Der AT- und Schenkelhalsschaftwinkel des Femur. Bücherei des Orthopäden, vol 10, Enke, Stuttgart

Kramps HA (1979) Einsatzmöglichkeiten der Ultraschalldiagnostik am Bewegungsappa-rat. Z Orthop 118: 355-364

Morscher E (1961) Die mechanischen Verhältnisse des Hüftgelenkes und ihre Beziehung zum Halsschaftwinkel und insbesondere zur AT des Schenkelhalses. Z Orthop 94: 375-394

Moulton A, Upadhyay SS (1982) A direct method of measuring femoral anteversion us-ing ultrasound. J Bone Joint Surg [Br.] 64 B 14

Rippstein J (1955) Zur Bestimmung der AT des Schenkelhalses mittels zweier Röntgen-aufnahmen. Z Orthop 86: 345-360

Wilson DJ (1984) Arthrosonography of the painful hip. Clin Radiol 35: 17-19

Knee Joint

Technique of Examination

In principle the knee joint should be examined in all areas that are accessible to sonographic imaging. Excellent longitudinal views are obtained by scanning above the patella at the center of the superior recess (suprapatellar pouch) and below the patella over the fat pad (Fig. 72). From those sites the transducer is moved laterally and medially to obtain parallel views of the condyles. The transducer is then rotated 90° and transverse scans are initiated proximally over the quadriceps muscle group with visualization of the vastus medialis, vastus lateralis, and the entire superior recess. Transverse scans are continued distal to the patella, delineating the infrapatellar space. The knee should always be examined in flexion so that the deformation of the fat pad, the downward excursion of the patella, and the narrowing of the superior recess can be observed. This is especially important when effusion is present so that the fluid displacement in the parapatellar spaces can be studied. In addition, flexion of the knee appears to produce a suction effect that draws fluid into the superior recess (Fig. 73).

When the anterior phase of the examination is completed, the patient is turned onto his stomach, and the medial and lateral condyles are scanned longitudinally from the posterior aspect beginning with a scan over the popliteal artery. Visualization of the epicondyles leads easily to misinterpretation because of their irregular structure, so scans should be performed between the epicondyles to remove this source of error.

The transducer then is rotated 90° for transverse scanning, as on the anterior side, proceeding in a proximal-to-distal direction. Scans through the intercondylar notch, joint space, and posterior inferior recess are particularly rewarding.

Dynamic examination of the knee joint is more difficult to perform with a linear array scanner, because flexion tends to raise the transducer from the skin and substantially reduce the contact area. This makes it necessary to use a standoff pad. On the other hand, the sector scanner with its small coupling surface is suitable even for dynamic examinations of the popliteal fossa (Fig. 74).

Compression of the thigh can be a helpful means of identifying the distended popliteal vein in close proximity to the popliteal artery.

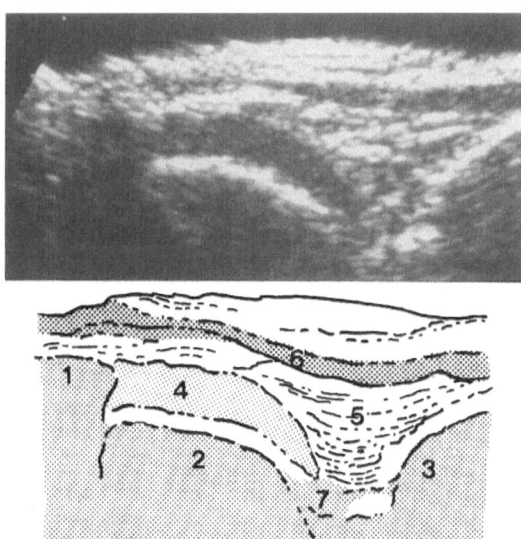

Fig. 72. Gonitis of the right knee in a patient with a 13-year known history of rheumatoid arthritis, infrapatellar longitudinal scan. **1** Patella, **2** femoral condyle, **3** tibia, **4** prefemoral inflammatory substrate, **5** infrapatellar fat pad, **6** patellar tendon, **7** joint space

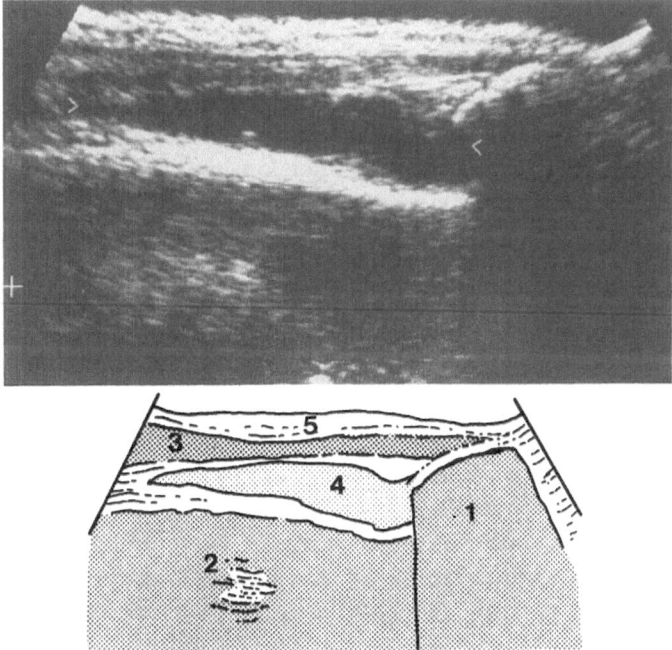

Fig. 73. Gonitis of the left knee with suprapatellar exudation in rheumatoid arthritis. **1** Patella, **2** femoral shaft, **3** patellar tendon, **4** superior recess with inflammatory substrate, **5** skin and subcutaneous tissue

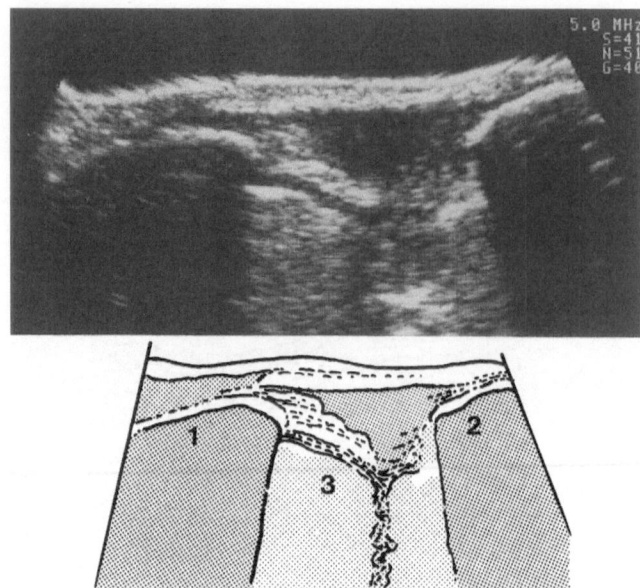

Fig. 74. Longitudinal infrapatellar scan showing a condylar prothesis in a 77-year-old man with seropositive rheumatoid arthritis. 1 Patella, 2 tibia, 3 prosthesis

Normal Sonographic Anatomy

The knee joint is examined first on static longitudinal and transverse scans in the recumbent patient. This is followed by a dynamic examination with passive joint motion. As Fig. 75 demonstrates, three longitudinal scans are of primary importance in the knee area:

Suprapatellar Longitudinal Scan

This scan demonstrates:
- the patella as an echogenic structure with a posterior acoustic shadow;
- the patellar tendon, whose echogenicity varies with the beam angle;
- the superior recess as a triangular area of nonhomogeneous echogenicity;
- the femoral surface as an echogenic structure with a posterior acoustic shadow;
- the pericondylar cartilage as an echo-free structure, generally no more than 2-3 mm thick, investing the condyle (if visible above the patella).

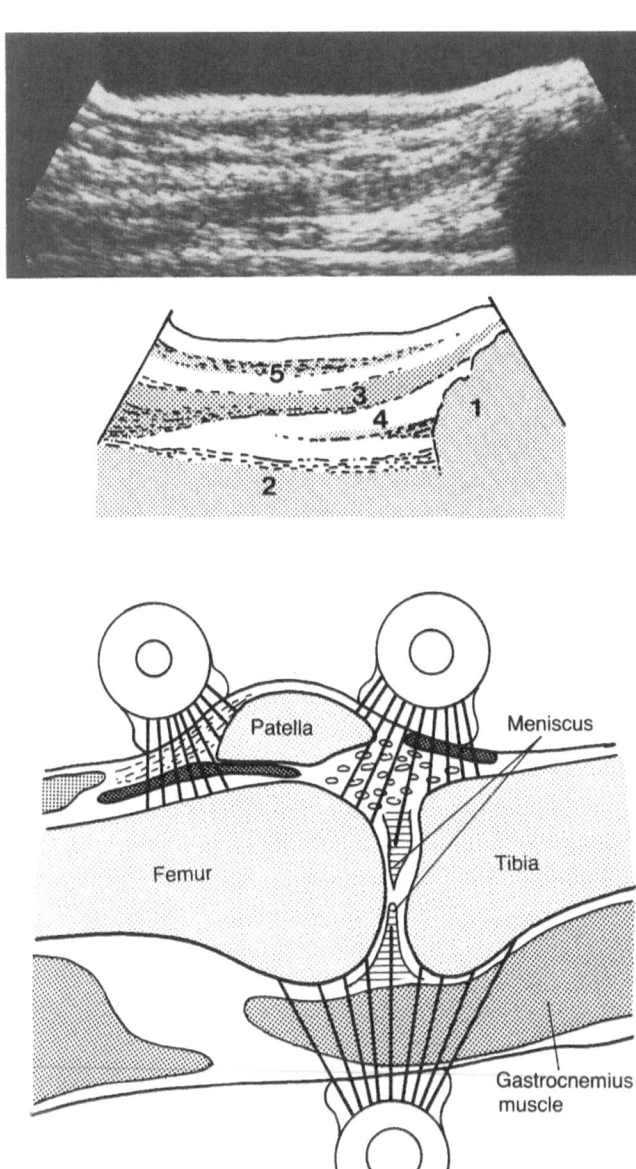

Fig. 75. Normal knee joint, longitudinal suprapatellar scan *(top).* **1** Patella, **2** femoral shaft, **3** patellar tendon, **4** superior recess, **5** skin and subcutaneous tissue. Diagram showing sites for longitudinal scanning of the knee joint *(bottom)*

Infrapatellar Longitudinal Scan

This scan demonstrates:
- the patella as an echogenic structure with a posterior acoustic shadow;
- the medial and lateral condyles, if visible below the patella;
- the anterior tibial margin and part of the tibial plateau as a band of bright echoes with posterior shadowing;
- the infrapatellar fat pad as an echogenic, nonhomogeneous structure lying below the patella and deforming with flexion;
- the prefemoral hyaline cartilage as a hypoechoic pericondylar band usually no more than 2–3 mm thick;
- the actual joint space bounded by the bony structures of the tibia and femur, seen most plainly during movement;
- the inferior recess bounded by the patellar tendon and the anterior surface of the tibia; it usually shows an irregular pattern of relatively high-level echoes (Figs. 76 and 77).

The meniscus cannot be defined as a homogeneous structure with a 5-MHz transducer, and lesions of the menisci are indistinguishable from normal findings.

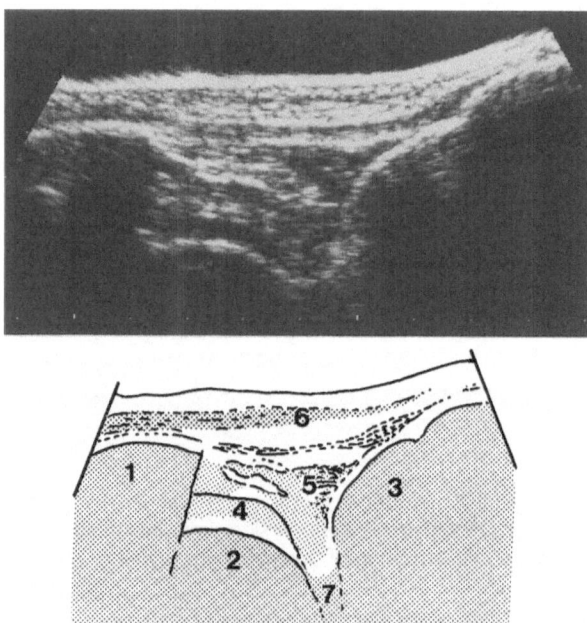

Fig. 76. Normal knee joint, longitudinal infrapatellar scan. **1** Patella, **2** femoral condyle, **3** tibia, **4** prefemoral hyaline cartilage, **5** infrapatellar fat pad, **6** patellar tendon, **7** joint space

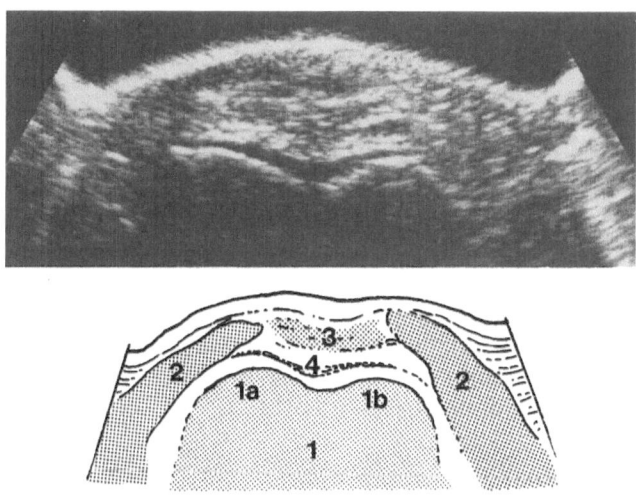

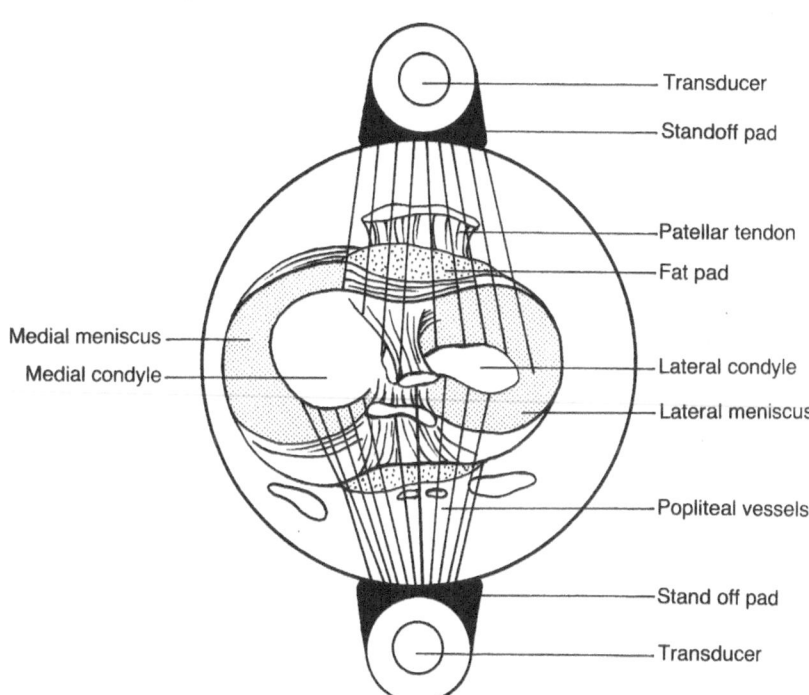

Fig. 77. Normal knee joint, transverse infrapatellar scan. **1** Femur, **1a** lateral femoral condyle, **1b** medial femoral condyle, **2** muscle, **3** patellar tendon (cut transversely), **4** intercondylar fossa. Diagram showing sites for transverse scanning of the knee *(bottom)*

Posterior Longitudinal Scan

- Both condyles appear as half- to three-quarter circles with associated acoustic shadows.
- The popliteal artery forms a "blinking" landmark at the medial border of the lateral condyle and is recognized by its echo-free lumen and pulsatile motion. The popliteal vein can be identified by compression of the thigh to induce distension.
- Pericondylar cartilage structures normal to the beam appear hypoechoic and generally no more than 3 mm thick (in adults).
- The joint capsule is usually divided by a faint fatty structure anterior to the popliteal artery. Ordinarily this fatty tissue can be clearly distinguished from the rest of the joint cavity (Figs. 78 a, b).

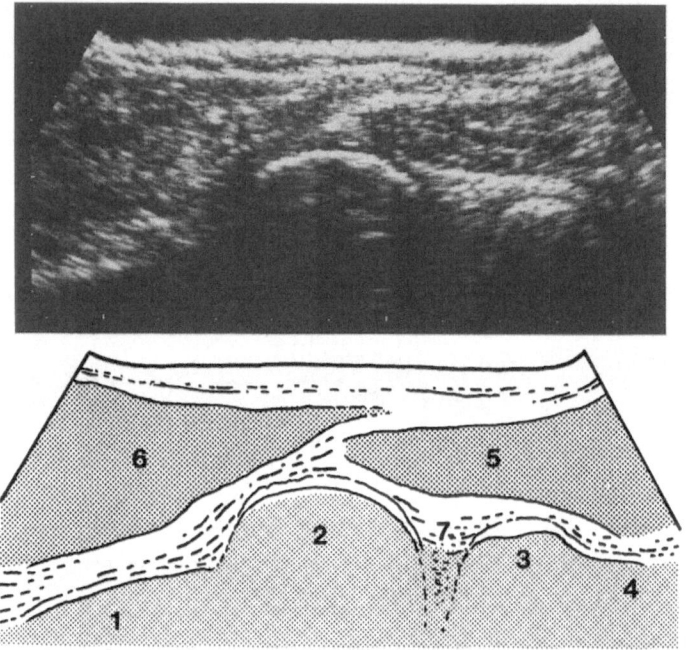

Fig. 78 a. Normal knee joint, posterior longitudinal scan over the lateral condyle. **1** Femoral shaft, **2** lateral femoral condyle, **3** tibial plateau, **4** tibial shaft, **5** gastrocnemius muscle, **6** biceps femoris muscle, **7** joint space

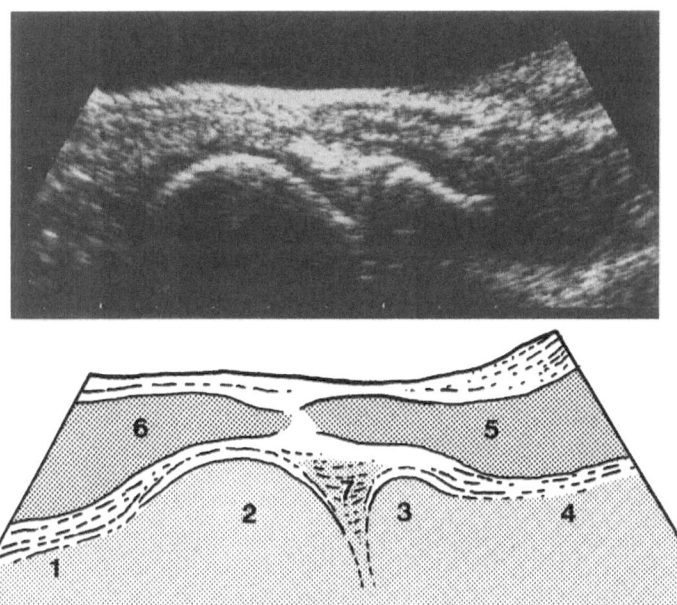

Fig. 78 b. Normal knee joint, posterior longitudinal scan over the medial condyle.
1 Femoral shaft, **2** medial femoral condyle, **3** tibial plateau, **4** tibial shaft, **5** gastrocnemius muscle, **6** semimembranosus muscle, **7** joint space

According to studies by C. Sohn and H. Gerngross, the meniscus can be visualized between the femur and tibia on the posterior longitudinal scan when a 7.5-MHz transducer is used. The authors state that any type of meniscal lesion disrupts the homogeneous echo pattern (Fig. 79a), with tears appearing as sharply defined nonhomogeneities (Fig. 79b) and degenerative changes typically appearing as smaller, less well defined areas that are generally multifocal. Sonographic evaluation of the menisci is still in its early stages, and further studies are needed to substantiate these initial results.

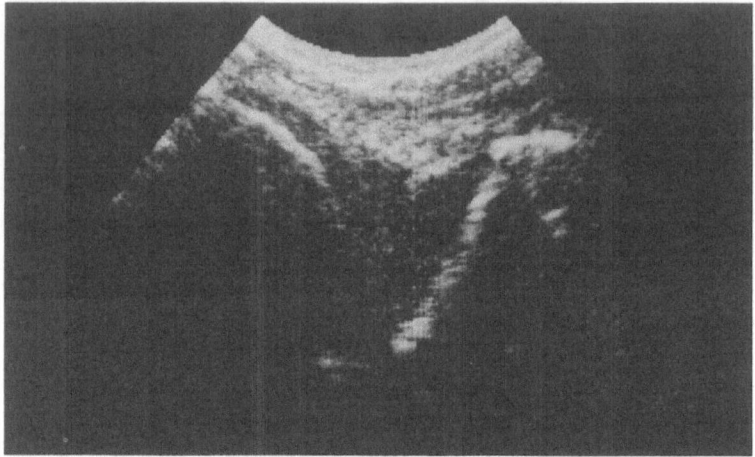

Fig. 79a. Normal finding: the posterior horn of the right lateral meniscus is seen as a triangular, homogeneous, moderately echogenic structure between the lateral condyle and the tibia

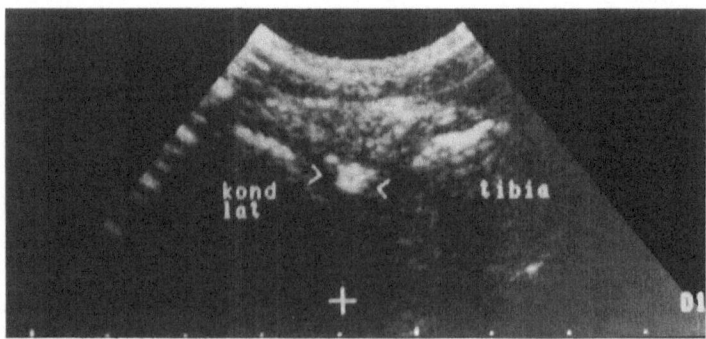

Fig. 79b. Pathologic finding: fresh meniscal tear, confirmed operatively. The tear presents as an area of intense echogenicity which can be traced over several planes

Interpretive Criteria

The presence of inflammatory change and/or effusion is characterized by enhanced sound transmission in the affected joint region. Specifically:
- A marked "thickening" of the inner capsule is seen in arthritis.
- Improved sound transmission intensifies the echo return from bone surfaces.
- Destructive bone changes create a discontinuity in the bony surface (Fig. 80).
- The muscles show increased echogenicity, and their contours are obscured.

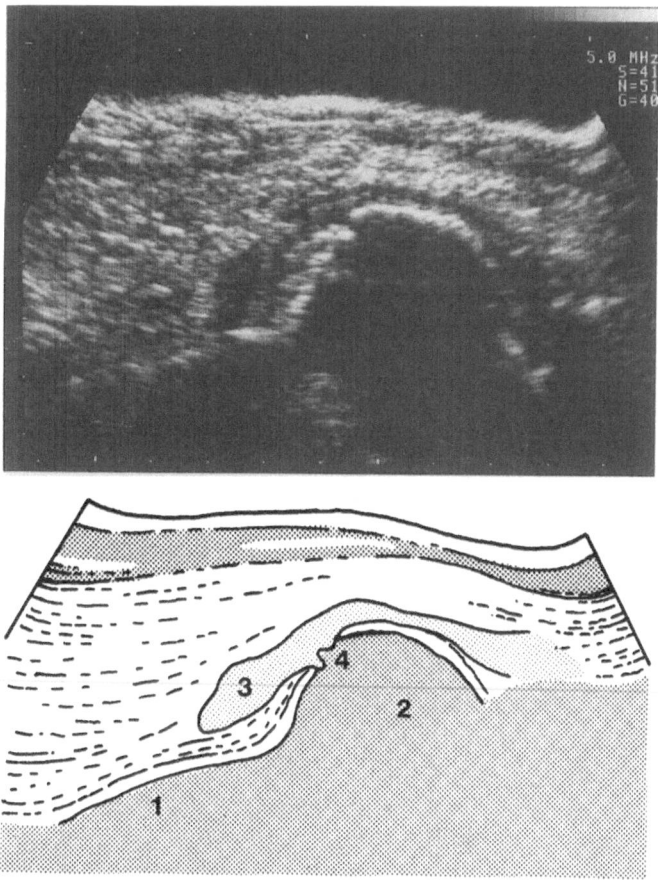

Fig. 80. Destructive gonitis in rheumatoid arthritis, posterior longitudinal scan over the lateral femoral condyle. **1** Femoral shaft, **2** lateral condyle, **3** inflammatory substrate, **4** osseous lesion

- The displacement of an effusion by palpation or joint motion is of particular importance. In flexion, for example, the superior recess is compressed ("squeezed out like a sponge") by pressure from the overlying patellar tendon (Fig. 81).

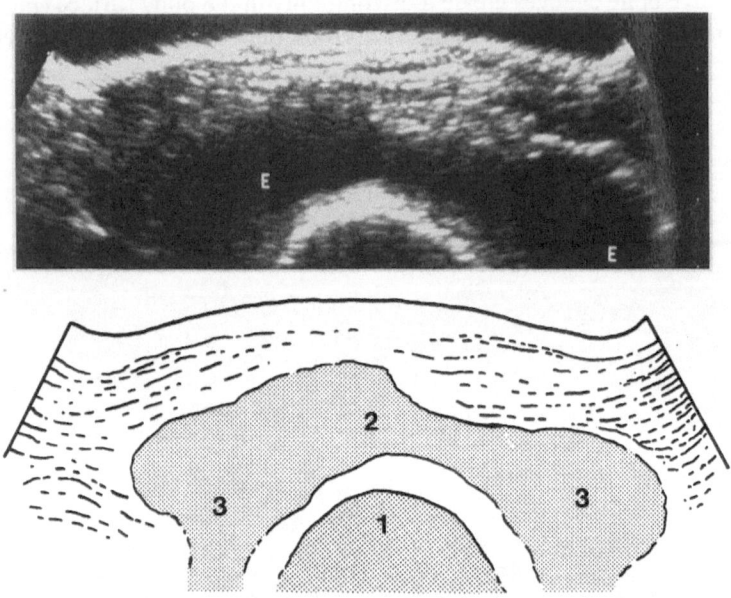

Fig. 81. Inflammatory exudate in the suprapatellar and parapatellar recesses leading to enhanced sound transmission with increased cortical echoes from the femoral shaft. **1** Femoral shaft, **2** suprapatellar exudate, **3** parapatellar exudate

Pathologic Conditions

The range of potential pathologic findings in the knee area is illustrated in
Fig. 82.

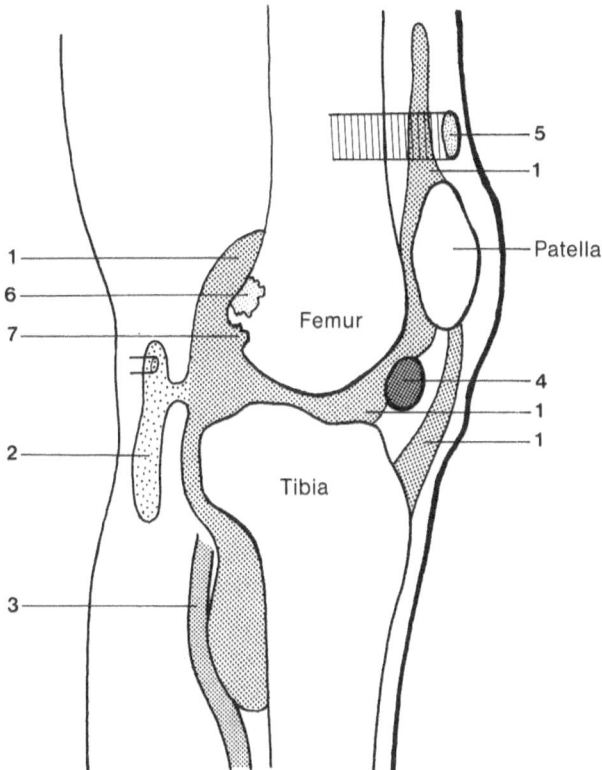

Fig. 82. Summary of sonographically detectable knee joint pathology. **1** Synovitis: suprapatellar, infrapatellar, and pericondylar in the popliteal fossa; **2** popliteal cyst; **3** enlarged posterior inferior recess with displacement of popliteal artery; **4** infrapatellar tumor; **5** suprapatellar calcification (e. g., osteochondritis dissecans); **6** defect formation;
7 erosion

Gonitis

We are unable to visualize inflammatory processes in all areas of the joint, but areas accessible to sonography can serve as windows through which the knee can be evaluated for inflammatory disease. These are, from the anterior aspect:

- the superior recess (Figs. 83 and 84) and
- the infrapatellar joint space with the inferior recess (Figs. 85 and 86);
  and from the posterior aspect:
- the medial and lateral pericondylar portions of the joint capsule (Fig. 87),
- the posterior joint space,
- the posterior inferior recess.

The anterior superior recess is particularly easy to locate and identifiy. It appears as a cigar-shaped, hypoechoic structure above the patella, showing biconvex enlargement in the presence of inflammatory disease. The excellent sound conduction through the recess causes the underlying femoral cortex to appear intensely echogenic.

Prefemoral inflammatory processes are also seen distal to the patella. They are characterized by infrapatellar thickening of the synovium, which appears as a hypoechoic structure surrounding the infrapatellar fat pad. Scans from the posterior aspect demonstrate the medial and lateral femoral condyles with their synovial investment. Occasionally, thickening of the chondro-osseous junction in the posterior superior recess may be seen as the only sign of incipient inflammation. Synovial thickening appears about the condyles, and the enhanced pericondylar sound conduction leads to increased echogenicity of the cortical bone, whose contours appear very pronounced. This makes it easier to recognize discontinuities associated with destructive bone changes. With the progression of inflammatory disease, fluid collection in the posterior joint space supervenes on the pericondylar changes and enhances the contours of the tibial plateau and posterior tibial margin. On the sonogram the dorsal synovitis assumes the shape of the Greek letter "tau" over the posterior joint space.

When the posterior inferior recess becomes distended, it creates a teardrop-shaped "sac" which clearly outlines the posterior tibial contour. This may cause displacement of the adjacent popliteal vessels, so elongation and compression of these vessels is sometimes observed as a direct consequence of the inflammatory mass effect (Fig. 88).

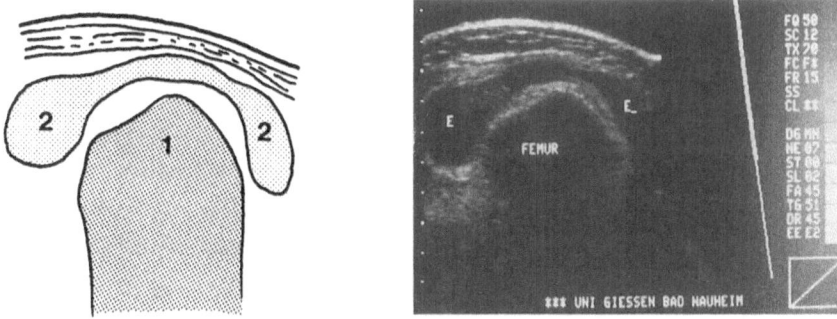

Fig. 83. Fifty-two year old man with rheumatoid arthritis, transverse suprapatellar scan showing collection of inflammatory exudate (**E**) in the parapatellar spaces. **1** Transverse section of femoral shaft with acoustic shadowing, **2** exudate-filled parapatellar spaces

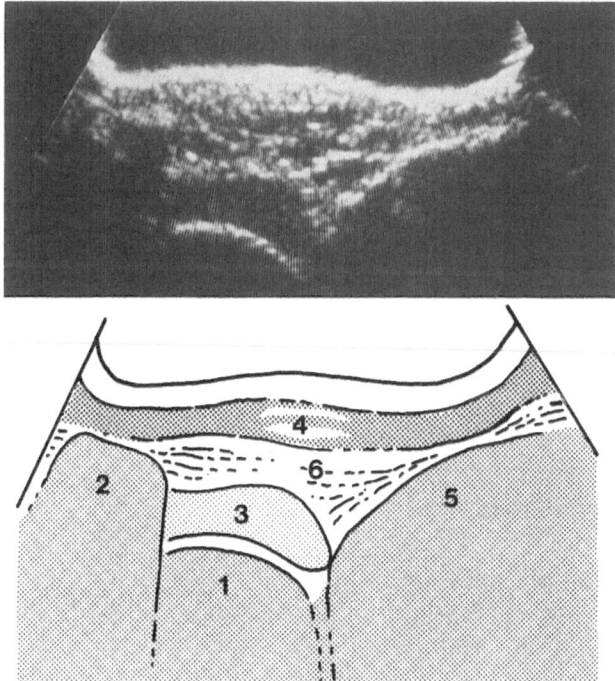

Fig. 84. Fifty-eight year old woman with seropositive rheumatoid arthritis, infrapatellar longitudinal scan. **1** Femoral condyle, **2** patella with acoustic shadow, **3** infrapatellar prefemoral inflammatory substrate, **4** patellar tendon, **5** tibia, **6** infrapatellar fat pad

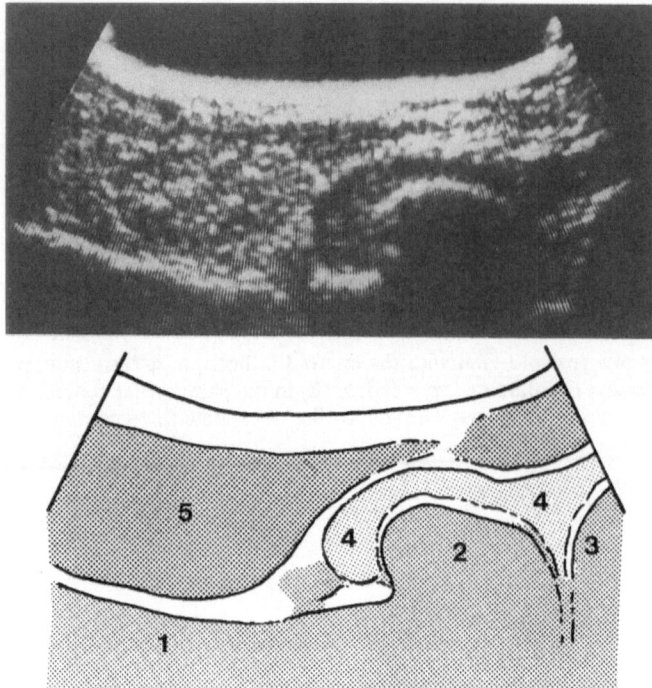

Fig. 85. Sixty-six year old woman with rheumatoid arthritis (proliferative-type synovitis by histology). **1** Femoral shaft, **2** lateral femoral condyle, **3** tibial plateau, **4** synovitis, **5** biceps femoris muscle

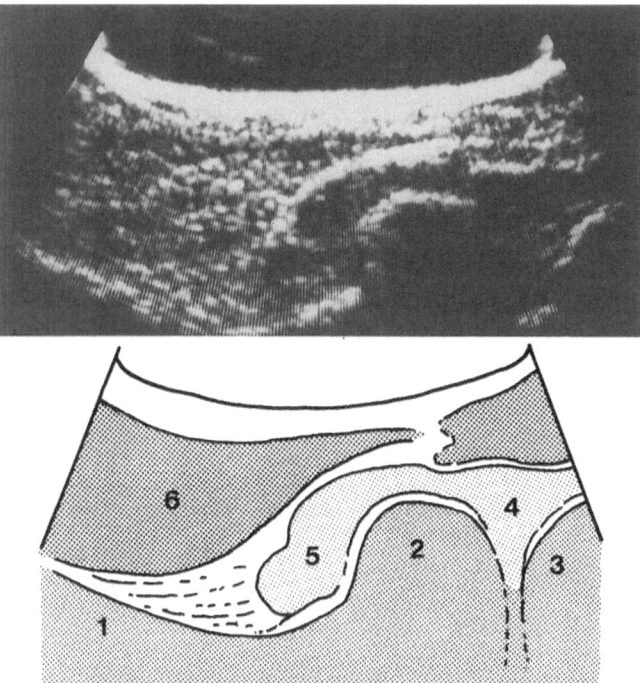

Fig. 86. Sixty-six year old woman with rheumatoid arthritis (proliferative-type synovitis by histology). **1** Femoral shaft, **2** lateral femoral condyle, **3** tibial plateau, **4** synovitis in posterior joint space, **5** synovitis over condyle and in paraosseous joint pouch, **6** biceps femoris muscle

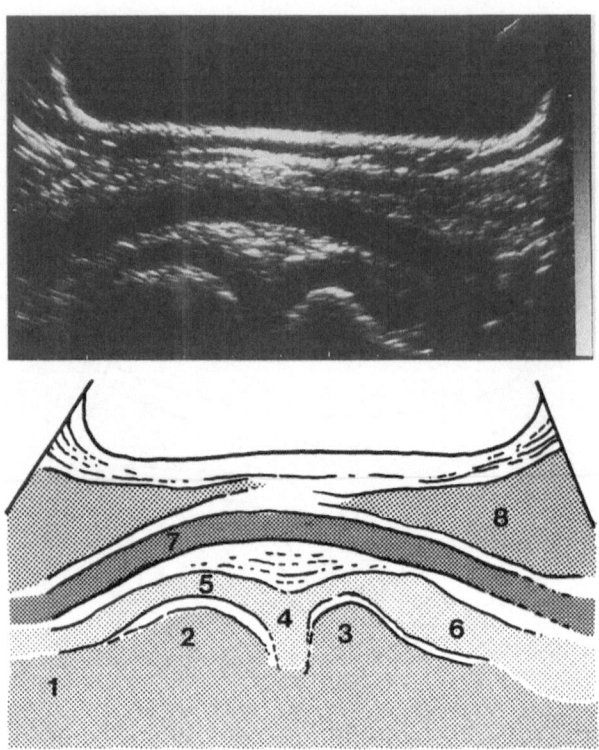

Fig. 87. Sixty-four year old woman with psoriatic arthritis, posterior longitudinal scan over the popliteal artery. **1** Femoral shaft, **2** femoral condyle, **3** upper tibia, **4** posterior joint space, **5** pericondylar inflammatory substrate, **6** inflammatory substrate in posterior inferior recess, **7** popliteal artery, **8** muscle

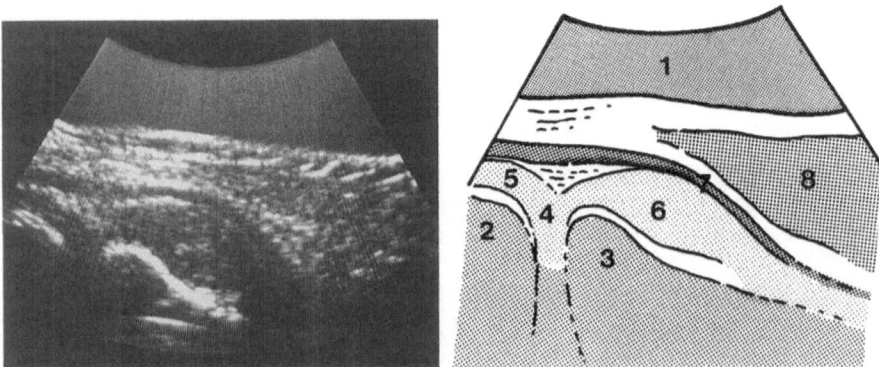

Fig. 88. Fifty year old woman with rheumatoid arthritis, inflammatory substrate in the enlarged posterior inferior recess compressing the popliteal artery and displacing it posteriorly. **1** Standoff pad, **2** femoral condyle, **3** upper tibia, **4** joint space, **5** pericondylar inflammatory substrate, **6** inflammatory substrate in enlarged posterior inferior recess, **7** popliteal artery, **8** muscle

Effusion

Effusion occur at typical sites determined by gravity and the position of the knee. Thus, in the recumbent patient the fluid collects in the parapatellar recesses. Joint motion changes the shape of the collection. Effusion show a variety of echo patterns ranging form hypoechoic to mixed with villus-like internal echoes in a hypoechoic fluid medium (Figs. 89 and 90).

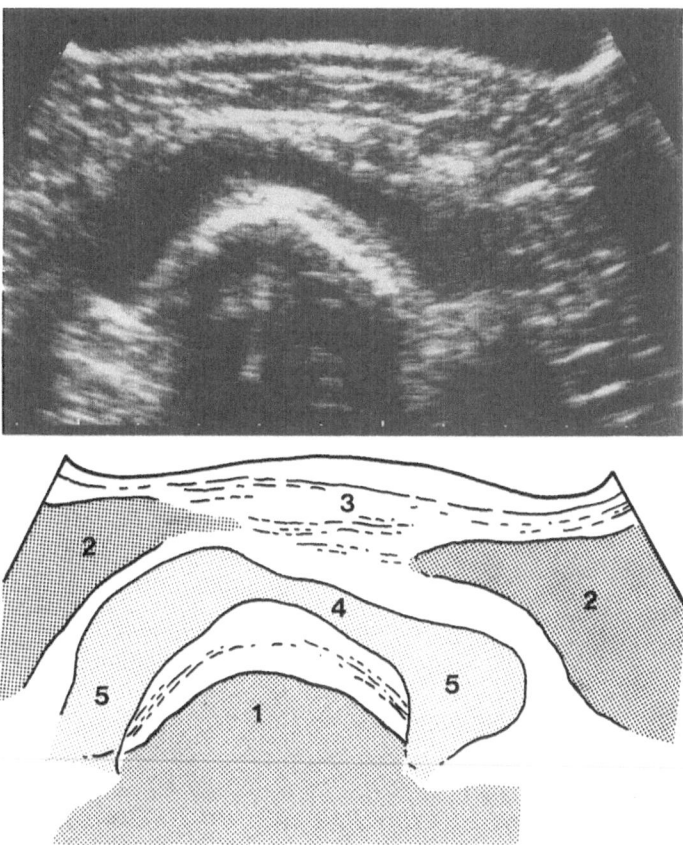

Fig. 89. Exudation in the suprapatellar and parapatellar recesses in active osteoarthritis, transverse suprapatellar scan. **1** Femoral shaft, **2** muscle, **3** patellar tendon, **4** exudate in superior recess, **5** exudate in parapatellar recesses

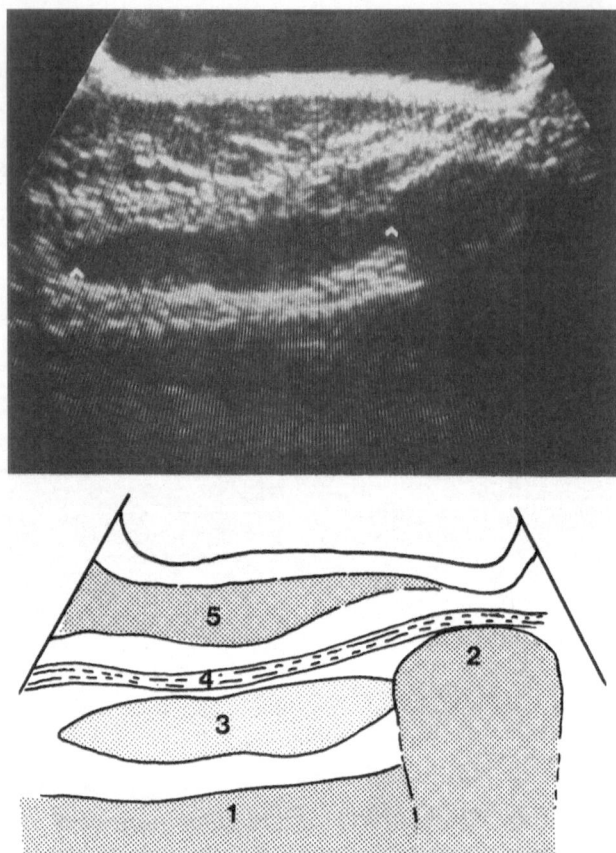

Fig. 90. Suprapatellar effusion, anterior longitudinal scan. **1** Femoral shaft, **2** patella with acoustic shadow, **3** fluid-filled superior recess, **4** patellar tendon, **5** skin and sub-cutaneous tissue

Popliteal Cysts

Extra-articular fluid collections in the popliteal fossa are very often named after W. M. Baker (Baker's cysts). This is historically incorrect, however, because the Irish surgeon Adams published a description of popliteal synovial cysts before Baker, and because Baker, in his second classic publication of 1885, described not only cystic lesions of the popliteal region that communicated with the joint but also cysts about other large joints such as the hip, ankle, shoulder, elbow, and wrist. Baker's name, then, could be applied with equal validity to any synovial cyst of a large joint.

Popliteal cysts, known variously as synovial cysts, hygromas, and "hernias of the knee," present as sharply defined lesions in the medial portion of the popliteal fossa. They are always extra-articular. Because of their location, they tend to spread distally and dissect between the heads of the gastrocnemius. A popliteal cyst is easily distinguished from surrounding muscle by its cystic echo pattern and smooth walls.

Popliteal cysts can vary considerably in their shape and echo characteristics, as the diagram on p. 104 illustrates. They occur in the setting of degenerative as well as inflammatory arthritis. It remains to be determined whether the echogenicity of the cyst (e. g., hyperechocity signifying a high fibrin content) may be helpful in establishing its origin (Figs. 91-96, see Fig. 82).

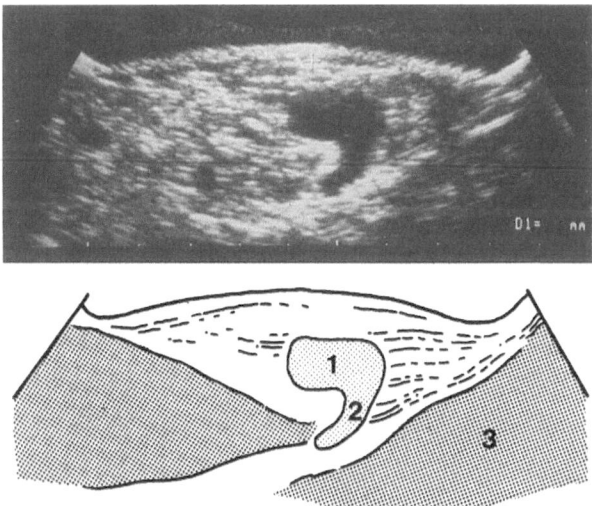

Fig. 91. Transversely cut synovial cyst in the popliteal fossa between the heads of gastrocnemius. **1** Popliteal cyst, **2** connecting channel, **3** muscle

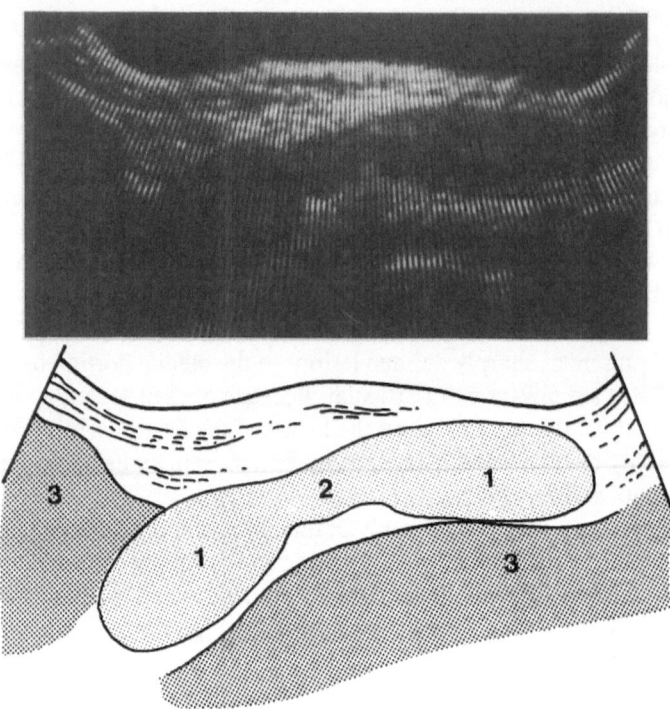

Fig. 92. Large hourglass-shaped popliteal cyst extending to the midcalf level, posterior longitudinal scan. **1** Popliteal cyst, **2** connecting channel, **3** muscle

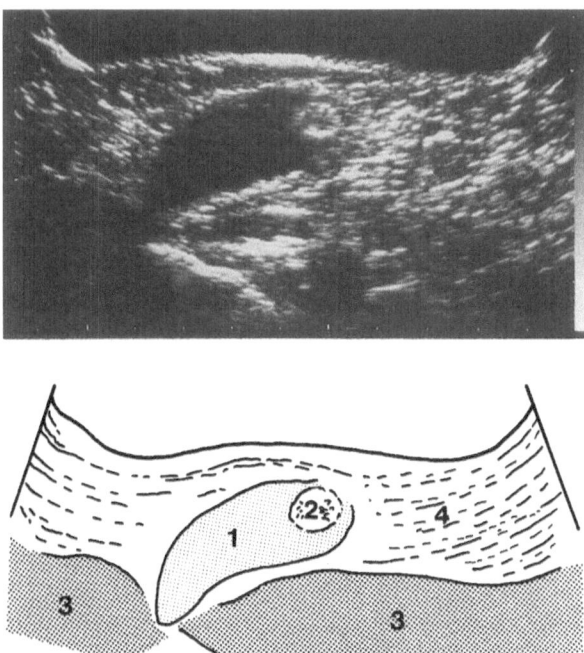

Fig. 93. Popliteal cyst at typical site containing a highly echogenic structure (bone sequestrum) which casts an acoustic shadow. **1** Popliteal cyst, **2** bone sequestrum, **3** muscle, **4** fibrofatty tissue

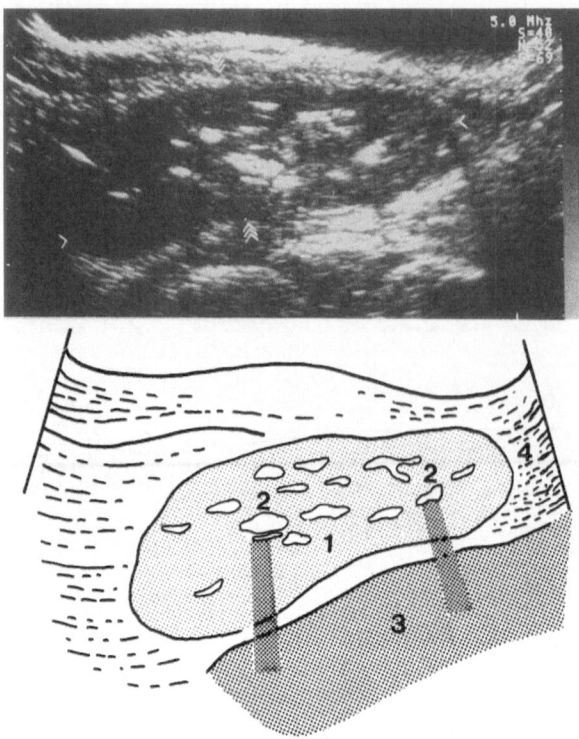

Fig. 94. Large popliteal cyst at typical site containing multiple reflectors (fibrin collections and calcifications). **1** Popliteal cyst, **2** calcium-dense structures with acoustic shadows, **3** muscle, **4** fibrofatty tissue

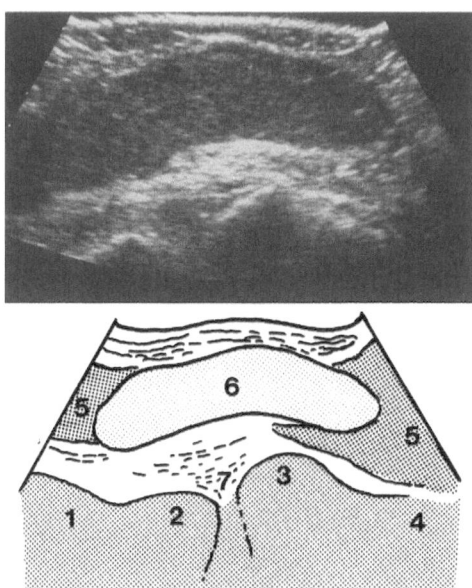

Fig. 95. Popliteal cyst in rheumatoid arthritis, posterior longitudinal scan over the right popliteal fossa. 1 Femoral shaft, 2 femoral condyle, 3 upper tibia, 4 tibial shaft, 5 muscle, 6 popliteal cyst with fine internal echoes from fibrin and debris, 7 joint space

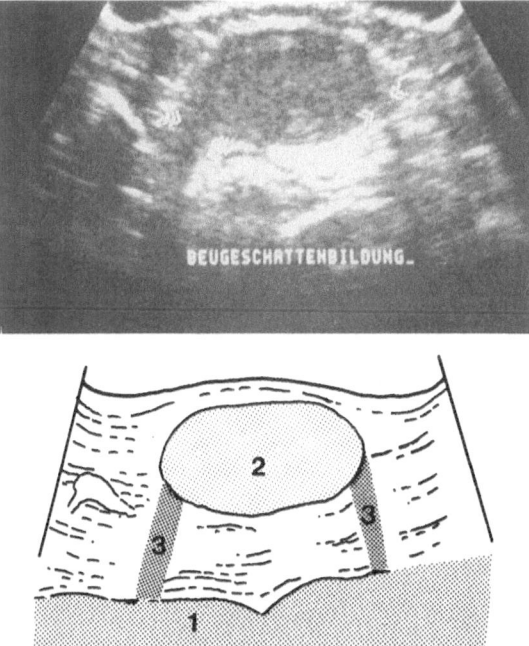

Fig. 96. Popliteal cyst in the right popliteal fossa with diffraction shadows. 1 Tibia, 2 popliteal cyst, 3 diffraction shadows. *Beugeschattenbildung:* Diffraction shadows

Shapes and Echo Patterns of Popliteal Cysts

oval

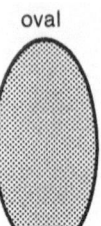

Wedge shaped

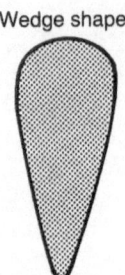

Hourglass shaped

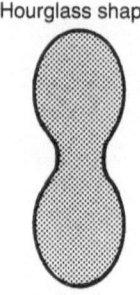

Round

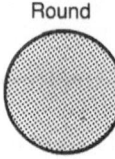

Egg shaped

Tubular

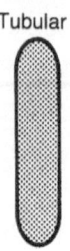

Hypoechoic

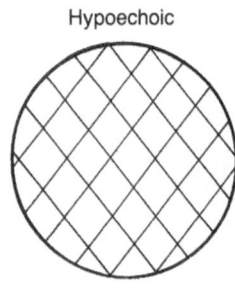

Hyperechoic

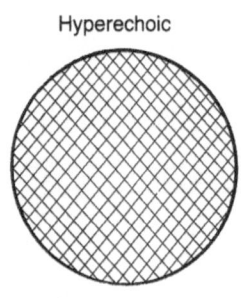

Mixed pattern

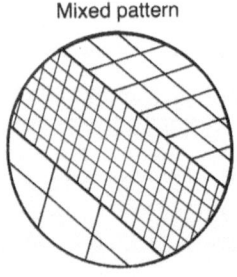

Complex pattern

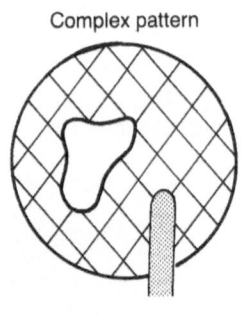

Echo-free areas

Echogenic structures
with acoustic shadows

Solid Tumors

Because arthrosonography is an indirect imaging technique, it cannot furnish a specific diagnosis for any given lesion. Thus, while sonography is able to detect a tumor in the knee area, it cannot provide a differential diagnosis of tumor type (Fig. 97).

Tumors appear as space-occupying lesions having a variable contour and variable echo pattern. They may lead to the following complications:

- displacement and compression of normal anatomic structures;
- deflection of blood vessels;
- sonographically detectable distant metastases (liver, pleura, lymph nodes, ascites).

Cysts are the most common mass lesions of the popliteal fossa. Mass effects are also produced by synovial proliferation, as noted earlier. In addition there are a great variety of benign and malignant tumors of the knee area, including:

1. *Benign tumors:* lipomas, fibromas, myxomas, angiomas, osteomas, xanthomatous giant cell tumors, synovial chondromatosis, pigmented villonodular synovitis.
2. *Malignant tumors:* malignant synovialomas with or without giant cells, metastases (especially from plasmacytoma and bronchogenic carcinoma).

A histologic or cytologic examination is necessary for a specific diagnosis of tumor type.

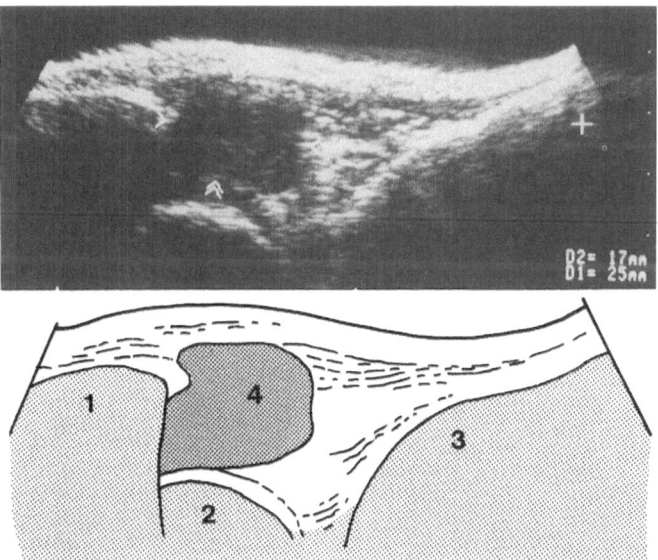

Fig. 97. Hypoechoic, relatively sharply marginated mass displacing the infrapatellar fat pad in the anterior joint space of the knee. Histology: benign giant cell tumor. **1** Patella, **2** femoral condyle, **3** tibia, **4** tumor

Meniscal Ganglion (Fig. 98)

This lesion appears as a hypoechoic structure near the base of the menisci. It is rounded, of variable size, and has relatively smooth margins. The cystoid nature of the lesion is evidenced by distal acoustic shadowing.

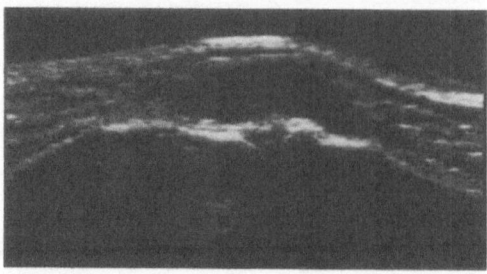

Fig. 98. Meniscal ganglion. Medial longitudinal scan shows an anechoic, relatively sharply marginated structure in the medial joint space of the knee

Vascular Changes

The entire course of the popliteal artery, including its origin from the femoral artery, is easily traced with ultrasound, and displacements of the vessel by mass lesions in the popliteal fossa are easily recognized. Besides mass lesions such as cysts and tumors, the vessel is commonly displaced or angulated by an enlarged and fluid-filled posterior inferior recess in the setting of inflammatory arthritis or osteoarthritis (exudation).

Sonographic evaluation of the knee area is indicated in all patients with a vascular disease of the lower leg. The sudden and unexpected distal extension of a popliteal cyst can incite an acute venous thrombosis or thrombophlebitis. This underscores the importance of knee sonography as an adjunct to the work-up of patients with lower leg edema. Popliteal cysts can also lead to vascular compression.

Arteriosclerotic changes produce irregularities in the wall of the popliteal artery, and these may or may not show acoustic shadowing. Most of these lesions are intensely echogenic, and some project into the vascular lumen. Dilatations and aneurysms of the popliteal artery are also found in this region and are identical to analogous lesions occuring elsewhere. A true popliteal aneurysm with complete dilatation of the vessel wall shows spontaneous luminal expansion with small echoes occupying at least a portion of the lumen. The latter finding signifies thrombosis (Fig.99).

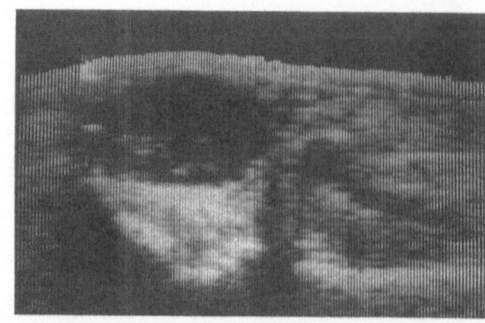

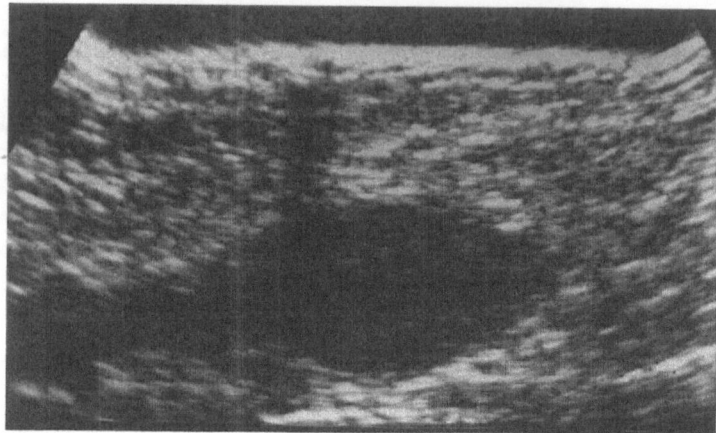

Fig. 99. a Aneurysm of the left popliteal artery: A smaller, true popliteal aneurysm is seen proximal to a larger aneurysm with pronounced thrombosis. (Scan taken with a Siemens Vidoson unit in 1979.) **b** Femoral aneurysm found above the right knee in a 62-year-old man with late-onset rheumatoid arthritis associated with advanced arterial occlusive disease. There is a marked fusiform dilatation of the femoral artery with thrombotic material outlining the vascular lumen: "sandwich" phenomenon. Longitudinal scan of the right femoral artery just above the popliteal fossa. **c** Schematic drawing

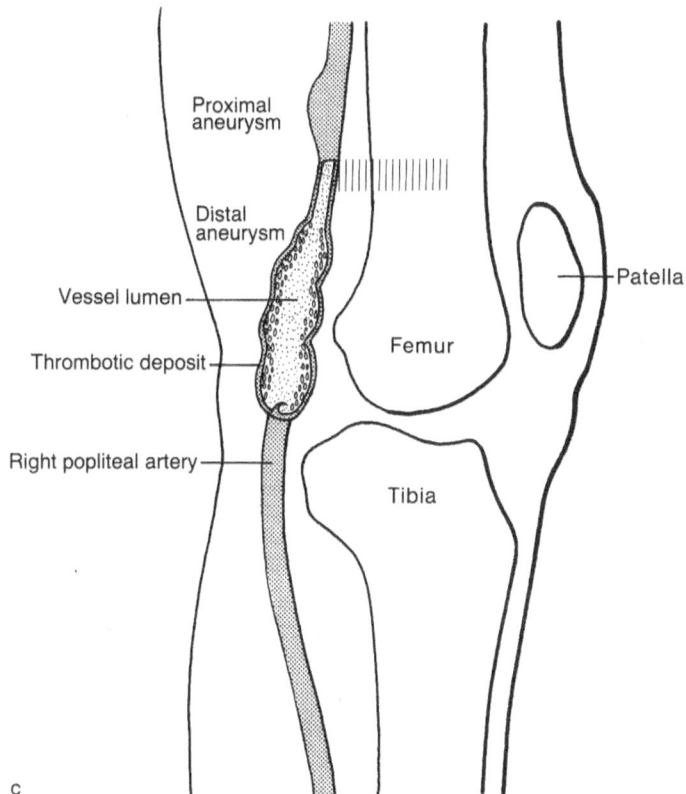

Proximal
aneurysm

Distal
aneurysm

Vessel lumen

Thrombotic deposit

Right popliteal artery

Femur

Tibia

Patella

c

Fig. 99 c

References

Adams M (1840) Chronic rheumatic arthritis of the knee joint. Dublin J Med Sci 27: 520–522

Aisen AM, McCune WJ, MacGuire A, Carson PL, Silver TM, Jafri SZ, Martel W (1984) Sonographic evaluation of the cartilage of the knee. Radiology 153 (3): 781–784

Ambanelli U, Manganelli P, Nervetti A, Urgolotti U (1976) Demonstration of articular effusions and popliteal cysts with ultrasound. J Rheumatol 3: 134

Baker WM (1877) Formation of synovial cysts in the leg in connection with disease of knee joint. St. Bartholomew's Hosp Rep 13: 245–261

Baker WM (1885) The formation of abnormal synovial cysts in connection with the joints. St. Bartholomew's Hosp Rep 21: 177–190

Baldassare AR, Auclair RJ, Carls GL, Zuckner J (1977) Dissecting popliteal cyst in a child with juvenile rheumatoid arthritis. J Rheumatol 4: 186–188

Barbaric ZL, Young LW (1972) Synovial cysts in juvenile rheumatoid arthritis. AJR 116: 655–660

Baumann D, Kremer H (1977) Arthrografie und Sonografie in der Diagnostik von Bakerzysten. ROFO 127 (5): 463–466

Bell JM, Ross FG, Mackenzie S, Goddard PR (1985) The swollen leg: ultrasonographic demonstration of non-thrombotic causes. Postgrad Med J 61 (711): 23–27

Braunstein EM, Silver TM, Martel W et al. (1981) Ultrasonographic diagnostis of extremity masses. Skeletal Radiol 6: 157

Brockmann WP, Wilmsdorff HV (1983) Gelenke mit Real-Time Sonographie des Körpers. In: Bückeler E, Friedmann G, Thelen H (eds) Real-time-Sonografie des Körpers. Thieme, Stuttgart

Bywaters EGL (1965) Editorial. The bursea of the body. Ann Rheum Dis 24: 215–218

Carpenter JR, Hattery RR, Hunder GG (1976) Ultrasound evaluation of popl. space: comparison with arthrographie and physical examination. Mayo Clin Proc 51: 498

Childress HM (1970) Popliteal cysts associated with undiagnosed posterior lesions of the medial meniscus. J Bone Joint Surg (Am) 52-A: 1487–1492

Cooperberg PL, Tsang IT, Truelove L (1978) Gray scale ultrasound in the evaluation of rheumatoid arthritis of the knee. Radiology 126: 759

Corbetti F, Schiavon F, Fiocco U, Angelini F, Gambari PF (1985) Unusual antefemoral dissecting cyst. Br J Radiol 58 (691): 675–677

DeAndrade JR, Grant C, Dixon AStJ (1965) Joint distension and reflex muscle inhibition in the knee. J Bone Joint Surg [Am] 47-A: 313–322

Derks WH, de Hooge P, van Linge B (1986) Ultrasonographic detection of the patellar plica in the knee. JCU 14 (5): 355–360

Dinham JM (1975) Popliteal cysts in children. The case against surgery. J Bone Joint Surg [Br] 57 B: 69–71

Dragonat P, claussen C (1980) Sonogr. Meniskusdarstellung. ROFO 133 (2): 185–187

Ernst J (1985) Ultraschalldiagnostik in der Rheumatologie. Aktuel Rheumatol 10: 35

Fedullo LM, Bonakdarpour A, Moyer Ra, Tourtellotte CD (1984) Giant synovial cysts. Skeletal Radiol 12 (2): 90–96

Fornage BD, Touche DH, Raguet M, Jacob M, Segal Ph (1982) Accidents musculaires du sportif. Nouv Press Med 11: 571

Fornage BD, Touche DH, Segal Ph, Rifkin MD (1983) Ultrasonography in the evaluation of muscular trauma. J Ultrasound Med 2: 549

Fornage BD, Rifkin MD, Touche DH, Segal Ph (1984) Sonography of the patellar tendon: preliminary observations. AJR 143: 179–182

Gagnier F, Taillan B, Bruneton JN, Bonnard JM, Denis F, Commandre F, Euller-Ziegler L, Ziegler G (1986) Three cases of pigment villonodular synovitis of the knee. Ultrasound and computed tomography findings. ROFO 145 (2): 227–228

Gebel M, Poor M, Feisel J, Wittenborg A (1977) Sonografie: Erste diagnostische Maßnahmen bei gelenkerkrankten Patienten mit den klinischen Zeichen der akuten Unterschenkelthrombose. In: Kratochwill A, Reinold E (eds) Ultraschalldiagnostik. Thieme, Stuttgart

Gebel M, Marisch KW, Green PG (1982) Problematik der ab. Transmissionssonografie und mögl. zukünftige Anwendungen

Gerber NJ, Dixon AStJ (1974) Synovial cysts and juxta-articular bone cysts (geodes). Semin Arthritis Rheum 3: 323–348

Gerber NJ, Bacon PA (1974) Popliteal cysts and synovial rupture in osteoarthrosis. Rheumatol and Rehab 13: 98–100

Gerber NJ (1981) Popliteale Synovialzysten (Bakerzysten): Selbständiges Krankheitsbild oder Symptom? Verh Dtsch Ges Rheumatol 7: 148

Gompels SM, Darlington LG (1979) Grey scale ultrasonography an arthrography in evaluation of popliteal cysts. Clin Radiol 30: 539

Green PS, Schaefer LF, Jones ED, Suarez JR (1974) A new high performance ultrasonic camera. In: Green PS (ed) Acoustical holography, Vol 5. Plenum, New York, p 493

Hammer M, Mielke H, Wagener P, Schwarzrock R, Giebel G (1986) Sonography and NMR imaging in rheumatoid gonarthritis. Scand J Rheumatol 15 (2): 157–164

Hermann G, Yeh HC, Lehr-Janus C, Berson Bl (1981) Diagnosis of popl. cysts: double-contrast arthrography and sonography. AJR 137 (2): 369–372

Hohle M, Lossner C, Hohle B (1986) (Initial experiences with sonography of the knee joint). Erste Erfahrungen mit der Sonographie des Kniegelenkes. Beitr Orthop Traumatol 33 (8): 394–402

Kaufmann RA, Towbin RB, Babcock DS, Crawford AH (1982) Arthrosonography in the diagnosis of pigmented villonoduar synovitis. AJR 139/2: 396–398

Kramps HA (1977) Ultraschall am Bewegungsapparat. In: Kratochwil A, Reinold E (eds) Ultraschalldiagnostik. Thieme, Stuttgart, p 259

Kremer H, Schierl W, Schattenkirchner M, Baumann D, Metz I, Zöllner N (1977) Sonogr. Diagnostik von Kniegelenkszysten. MMW 119: 1183–1186

Kremer H, Röder K, Brettel H, Dobrinski W, Scherg C, Waidelich W, Zöllner N (1981) Transmissionssonografische Diagnostik der Extremitäten. In: Kratochwil A, Reinold E (eds) Ultraschalldiagnostik, Drei-Länder-Treffen, Graz. Thieme, Stuttgart

Laajam MA (1985) Synovial rupture complicating Brucella arthritis. Br J Rheumatol 24 (2): 191–193

Marhoffer W, Sattler H (1985) Zur Wertigkeit der Arthrosonographie vor und nach Synovektomie: Möglichkeiten der sonographischen Synovialitisdiagnostik. Ultraschalldiagnostik 85. Thieme, Stuttgart, p 644

Meire HB, Lindsay DJ, Swinson DR, Hamilton EBD (1974) Comparison of ultrasound and positive contrast arthrography in the diagnosis of popliteal and calf swelling. Ann Rheum Dis 33: 221

Müller-Brodmann W, Goebel KM (1982) Ultraschalldiagnostik entzündlicher Kniegelenkserkrankungen. Dtsch Med Wochenschr 107: 1400

Ramach W, Kratochwil A (1977) Die Ultraschalldiagnostik in der Orthopädie. In: Kratochwil A, Reinold E (eds) Ultraschalldiagnostik. Wien, Thieme, Stuttgart

Rautschning W (1979) Popliteal cyst and the relation to the gastrocnemio-semimembranosus-bursa. Studies on the surgical and functional anatomy. Acta Orthop Scand [Suppl]

Rauschning W, Lindgren PG (1979) Popliteal cysts (Baker's cyst) in adults. I. Clinical and roentgenological results of operative excision. Acta Orthop Scand 50: 583–591

Rauschning W (1980) Popliteal cysts (Baker's cysts) in adults. I. Capsuloplasty with and without a predicte graft. Acta Orthop Scand 51: 547–555

Rudikoff JC, Lynch JJ, Philipps E, Clapp PR (1976) Ultrasound diagnosis of Baker cyst. JAMA 235: 1054–1055

Röhr E (1985) (Experimental studies on the sonographic image of the cruciate ligament). Experimentelle Untersuchungen zur sonographischen Darstellung der Kreuzbänder. ROFO 143 (4): 467–468

Röhr E (1985) (Sonographic imaging of the posterior cruciate ligament). Die sonographische Darstellung des hinteren Kreuzbandes. Röntgenblätter 38 (12): 377–379

Sattler H, Gerhold H (1983) Die systematische Untersuchung des Knies mittels Ultraschall. In: Lutz H (ed) Ultraschalldiagnostik 83. Thieme, Stuttgart, p 527

Sattler H (1984) Was bietet die Sonographie in der Diagnostik der rheumatoiden Arthritis (chronische Polyarthritis). Ultraschalldiagnostik 84. In: Judmaier G, Fronmhold H, Kratochwil A (eds) Thieme, Stuttgart, p 246

Sattler H, Gerhold H (1984) Die Arthrosonographie – ein neues zusätzliches bildgebendes Verfahren in der Erfassung von Erkrankungen des Kniegelenkes. Z Rheumatol 43:160

Sattler H (1986) Die sonographische Erfassung eines Riesenzelltumors im Kniegelenk. Ultraschall Klin Prax I (I)-52: 43

Sattler H (1986) Die Arthrosonographie des Kniegelenkes bei rheumatoider Arthritis. Ultraschall Klin Prax I (2)-106: 99

Sohn C, Gerngroß H, Bähren W, Danz B (1987) Meniskussonographie – Alternative zur invasiven Meniskusdiagnosik?, Dtsch Med Wschr 112: 581–584

Sohn C, Gerngroß H, Bähren W, Swobodnik W (1987) Sonographie des Meniskus und seiner Läsionen, Ultraschall 8, 32–36

Sundermeyer R, Stolle E, Sattler H (1985) Sonographische Kniegelenksdiagnostik im Vergleich mit anderen bildgebenden Verfahren. In: Otto RC, Schnaars P (eds) Ultraschalldiagnostik 85. Thieme, Stuttgart, p 656

Seltzer SE, Finberg HJ, Weissmann BN (1978) Arthrosonography: technique, sonographic anatomy and pathology. Invest Radiol 126: 759

Seltzer SE, Finberg HJ, Weissmann BN (1979) Arthrosonography: grey scale ultrasound evaluation of the shoulder. Radiology 132: 467

Seltzer S, Finberg W, Weissmann B (1980) Arthrosonography – technique, sonographic anatomy, and pathology. Invest Radiol 15: 19

Steiger U, Wieser C, Zinn WM (1967) Synovialcysten und -rupturen des Kniegelenks. Schweiz Med Wochenschr 97: 1212–1215

Upadhyay SS, Moulton A, Burwell RG (1985) Biological factors predisposing to traumatic posterior dislocation of hip. A selection process in the mechanism of injury. J Bone Joint Surg [Br] 67 (2): 232–236

Woltering H (1985) (Ultrasonic diagnosis in orthopedics). Ultraschalldiagnostik in der Orthopädie. Z Orthop 123 (3): 416–419

Wyld PJ, Dawson KP, Chisholm RJ (1984) Ultrasound in the assessment of synovial thickening in the hemophilic knee. Aust NZ J Med 14 (5): 678–680

Zatz LM (1975) Initial clinical evaluations of a new ultrasonic camera. Radiology 117: 399

Zeymüller K, Kratochwil A (1975) Ultraschalldiagnostik bei Knochen- und Weichteiltumoren. Wien Klin Wochenschr 87: 397–398

Zuinen C, Carlier L, Gaudissart JL (1980) L'echotomographie en traumatologie musculaire. Medecine du Sport 54: 379

Ankle Joint

Technique of Examination

With the patient supine, longitudinal and transverse ankle scans are performed using a concave standoff pad at the junction of the lower leg and the dorsum of the foot. The ankle and subtalar joints are moved actively or passively during the examination.

The patient is then turned to the prone position, and posterior scans are obtained with the feet hanging over the end of the couch. A longitudinal scan is performed over the Achilles tendon while the ankle joint is moved by the examiner's free hand.

Normal Sonographic Anatomy

The ankles are examined on longitudinal and transverse planes anterior and posterior to the ankle and subtalar joints.

Anterior Longitudinal Scan over the Dorsum of the Foot

This scan demonstrates:
- the *tibia* and *talus* as bands of bright echoes with distal shadowing;
- the *navicular bone* (on medial scan).

The tendons of extensor hallucis longus and extensor digitorum longus are seen overlying the bony structures. These longitudinal structures may appear hyperechoic or hypoechoic, depending on the incidence angle of the beam ("wandering echo" phenomenon, q.v.). The joint capsule usually appears as a thin, hypoechoic zone over the ankle and subtalar joint spaces and is easily identified during joint motion.

- *Fatty tissue:* The extensor tendons and bony structures are separated by a fatty tissue layer of variable thickness and echogenicity which changes shape during passive joint motion (Fig. 100).

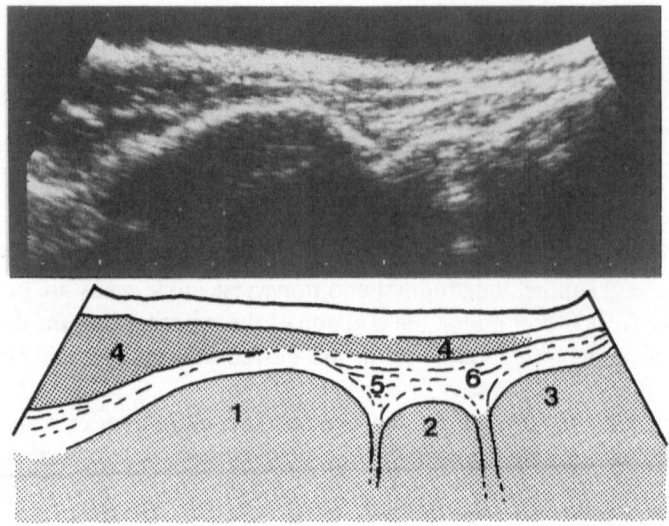

Fig. 100. Normal ankle and subtalar joints, longitudinal scan over the dorsum of the foot. **1** Tibia, **2** talus, **3** navicular bone, **4** extensor digitorum longus, **5** ankle joint space, **6** subtalar joint space

Posterior Longitudinal Scan

The area behind the tibia is also examined on longitudinal and transverse sections. Longitudinal scans just behind the Achilles tendon are particularly rewarding, though only a very small coupling surface is available in that region. The following structures can be identified (Figs. 101 and 102):

- The Achilles tendon is hyperechoic where perpendicular to the ultrasound beam, otherwise hypoechoic. The "wandering echo" phenomenon is plainly seen as the beam is swept over the tendon (Fig. 103).
- Subachilleal fat: Below the Achilles tendon is an area of fatty tissue with varying echogenicity. It contains the subachilleal bursa, which is clearly defined only when altered by disease.
- Posterior surface of tibia: Intense echoes along the tibial cortex mark its posterior surface.
- The posterior surface of the talus, also appearing as a line of bright echoes.

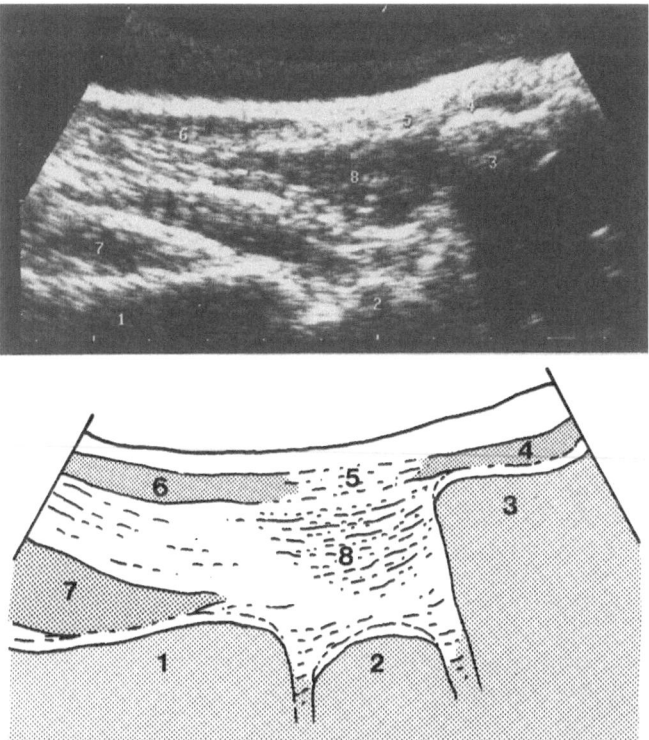

Fig. 101. Normal posterior ankle and subtalar joints, longitudinal scan over the Achilles tendon. **1** Tibia, **2** talus, **3** calcaneus, **4** insertion of Achilles tendon, **5** hyperechoic part of Achilles tendon, **6** hypoechoic part of tendon, **7** flexor digitorum longus and flexor hallucis longus, **8** subachilleal fat

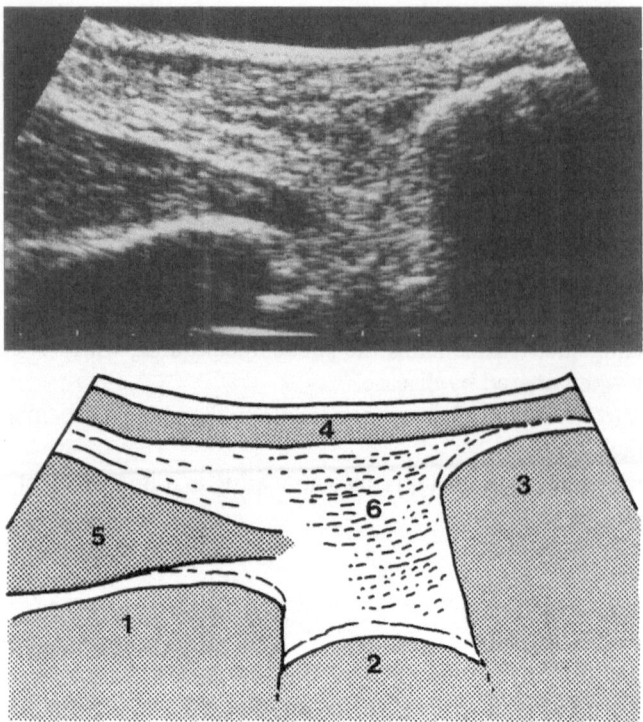

Fig. 102. Normal appearance of the ankle and subtalar joints, longitudinal scan over the Achilles tendon. **1** Tibia, **2** talus, **3** calcaneus, **4** Achilles tendon, **5** flexor digitorum longus and flexor hallucis longus, **6** subachilleal fat and connective tissue

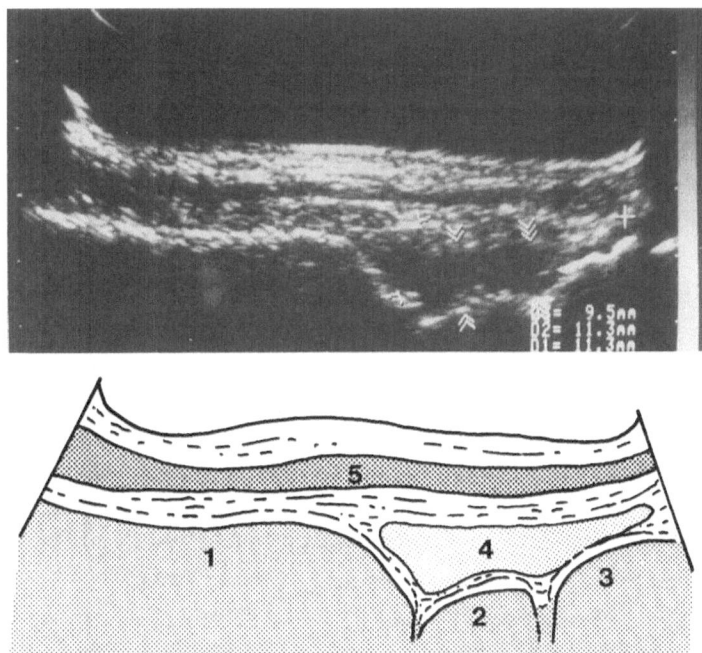

Fig. 103. Involvement of the ankle and subtalar joints in rheumatoid arthritis, longitudinal scan over the dorsum of the foot. **1** Tibia, **2** talus, **3** navicular bone, **4** inflammatory substrate, **5** muscle

- The calcaneus extends to the upper border of the image. Hypoechoic structures on the posterior surface of the calcaneus represent the normal Achilles tendon insertion.
- The ankle and subtalar joint spaces appear above and below the posterior border of the talus. They are seen most plainly during motion.
- The flexor hallucis longus and flexor digitorium longus form a hypoechoic structure that presents a regular echo pattern just behind the posterior surface of the tibia and changes shape during motion.

The muscle mass behind the tibia increases as the beam is moved proximad along the posterior tibial border. The capsule of the ankle and subtaler joints appears only as a very fine hypoechoic structure above the true joint space and in normal cases is virtually indistinguishable from surrounding fat and connective tissue.

Interpretive Criteria

Inflammatory processes alter sound conduction patterns about the ankle joint. Signs include thickening of the joint capsule, increased echogenicity of bone surfaces, enhanced delineation of the joint space, and increased sonodensity of hypertrophied muscles.

Pathologic Conditions

Arthritis

Exudative and proliferative processes in the synovium of the ankle or subtalar joint cause a pronounced "demarcation" of the joint space with a hypoechoic, sharply marginated mass apposing to the bone surfaces. The joint spaces, which normally are difficult to define even with motion, become sharply delineated by the sonoconductive inflammatory substrate (Figs. 104–106).

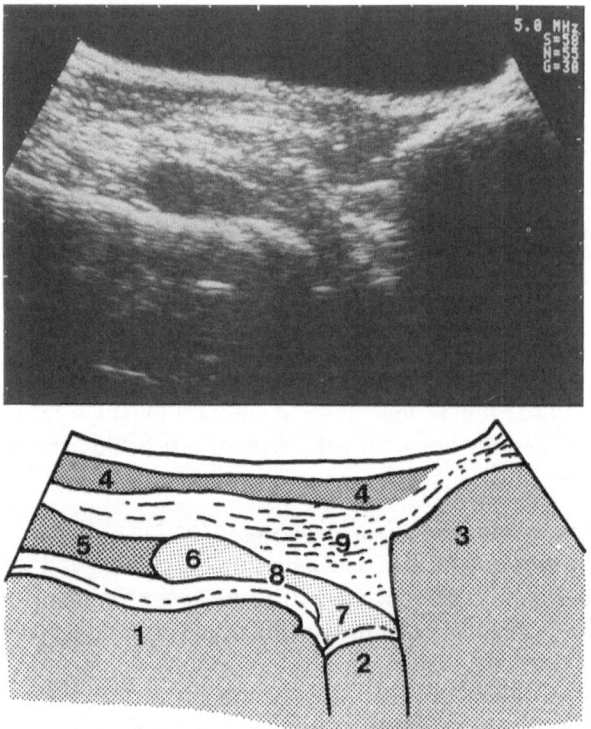

Fig. 104. Posterior ankle involvement in a 68-year-old woman with rheumatoid arthritis, longitudinal scan over the Achilles tendon. **1** Tibia, **2** talus, **3** calcaneus, **4** Achilles tendon, **5** flexor digitorum longus and hallucis longus, **6** synovial cyst, **7** inflammatory substrate, **8** connecting channel, **9** subachilleal fat and connective tissue

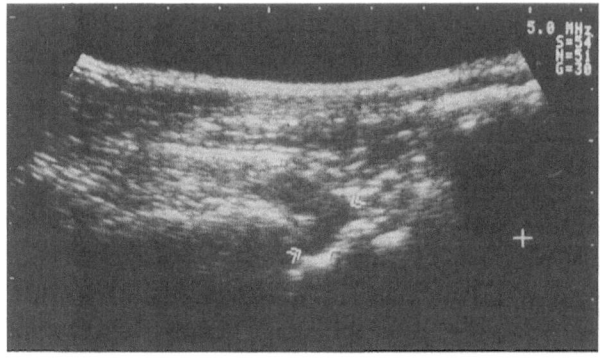

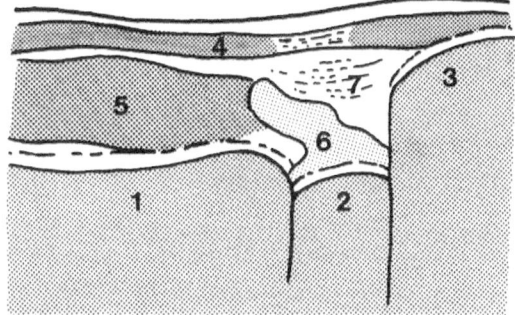

Fig. 105. Posterior ankle involvement in rheumatoid arthritis. **1** Tibia, **2** talus, **3** calcaneus, **4** Achilles tendon, **5** flexor digitorum longus and hallucis longs, **6** inflammatory substrate, **7** subachilleal fat and connective tissue

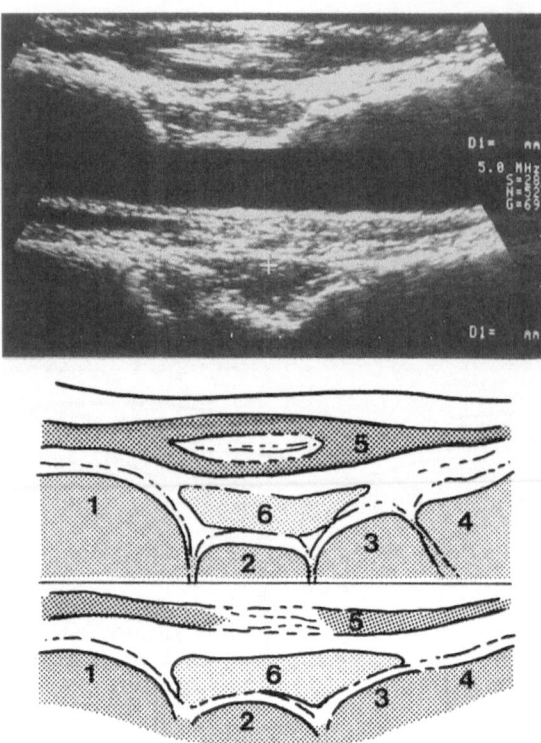

Fig. 106. *Upper panels:* Tenosynovitis of extensor digitorum longus tendon and moderate carpal arthritis, longitudinal scan over the ankle and subtalar joints. **1** Tibia, **2** talus, **3** navicular, **4** medial cuneiform, **5** tenosynovitis of extensor digitorum longus, **6** inflammatory substrate. *Lower panels:* Inflammatory change in the ankle and subtalar joints without tenosynovitis. **1** Tibia, **2** talus, **3** navicular, **4** medial cuneiform, **5** normal-appearing tendons of extensor digitorum longus, **6** inflammatory substrate

Tenosynovitis

The affected tendon appears as a central, hyperechoic structure within a tubular, hypoechoic sheath. This pattern has been likened to a "light road marking on dark asphalt." Because the tendons of extensor hallucis longus and extensor digitorum longus are well separated from the joint capsule by a layer of connective tissue and fat, tenosynovitis is easily differentiated from synovitis (see Fig. 106).

Bursitis

Subachilleal bursitis occuring in isolation or in the setting of other inflammatory disease is characterized by a sharply defined, hypoechoic mass with faint acoustic shadowing below the Achilles tendon. Experience has shown that the bursitis can be clearly distinguished from surrounding fatty tissue only when the volume of the bursa is markedly increased (Fig. 107).

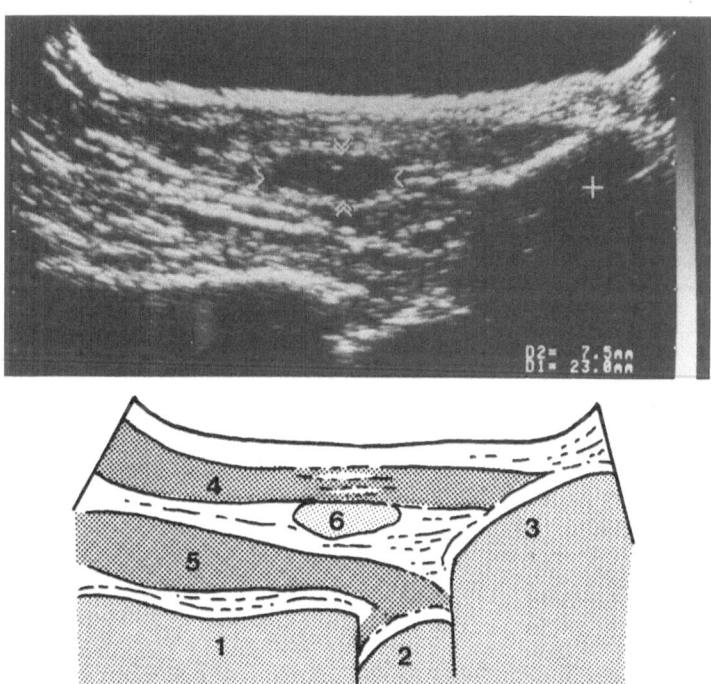

Fig. 107. Subachilleal bursitis, longitudinal scan over the Achilles tendon. 1 Tibia, 2 talus, 3 calcaneus, 4 Achilles tendon, 5 flexor hallucis longus and flexor digitorum longus, 6 inflammatory substrate in subachilleal bursa

Synovial Cysts

Any joint inflammation may be accompanied by the escape and collection of fluid in the extra-articular space. In the ankle, cysts of this kind appear below the flexor hallucis and brevis muscles directly over the tibial margin, presenting as oval structures with distal acoustic enhancement of the bone surface. Needle aspiration under sonographic guidance easily confirms the cystic nature of the lesion. The posterior longitudinal scan may demonstrate the channel along the posterior tibial border by which the synovial cyst communicates with the ankle joint (Fig. 108).

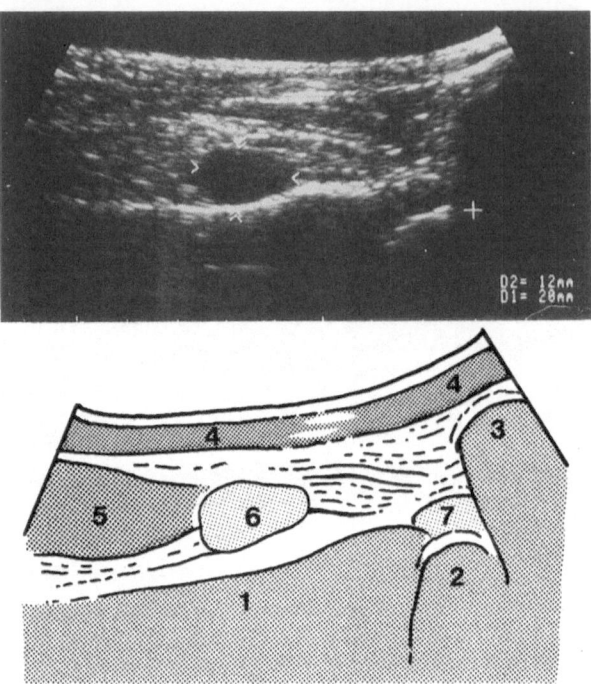

Fig. 108. Posterior ankle involvement in rheumatoid arthritis with a subachilleal synovial cyst, longitudinal scan over the Achilles tendon. **1** Tibia, **2** talus, **3** calcaneus, **4** Achilles tendon, **5** flexor hallucis longus and flexor digitorum longus, **6** synovial cyst, **7** inflammatory substrate

References

Mayer R, Wilhelm K, Pfeifer KJ (1984) Sonographie der Achillessehnenruptur. Digital Bilddiagn 4: 185

Reinherz RP, Zawada SJ, Sheldon DP (1986) Recognizing unusual tendon pathology at the ankle. J Foot Surg 25 (4): 278-283

Sattler H, Harland U, Marhoffer W (1985) Die Arthrosonographie des oberen und unteren Sprunggelenkes - Grenzen und Möglichkeiten. In: Otto RCH, Schnaars P (eds) Ultraschalldiagnostik 85. Thieme, Stuttgart, p 650

Sonography of the Soft Tissues

Technique of Examination

The ultrasound examination is preceded by a clinical examination which identifies the region of interest that is to be evaluated for sonographic change.

The first step in the sonographic examination is to establish the exact topography of the structure of interest. General or survey views are dispensed with. If it proves difficult to distinguish between closely adjacent anatomic structures, this can be aided by dynamic techniques. The alternate tensing of antagonistic muscle groups and the passive movement of joints, fingers, or toes will make it easier to appreciate topographic relationships (Fig. 109). In addition, linear movements and angulations of the transducer will give the examiner an impression of the size and relative position of pathologic structures.

Structural abnormalities in the soft tissues should always be imaged on at least two planes to avoid misinterpretation due to artifacts. If the changes involve tendons or muscles, combined longitudinal and transverse scanning is recommended.

The concurrent visualization of adjacent joint structures, deeper bony structures, or adjacent blood vessels is helpful for providing later spatial orientation in the documented image.

Bony structures yield intense surface echoes and can be evaluated only for superficial changes. Even a greatly thinned cortex is intensely echogenic and will prevent the evaluation of underlying structures (e.g., in patients with juvenile bone cysts).

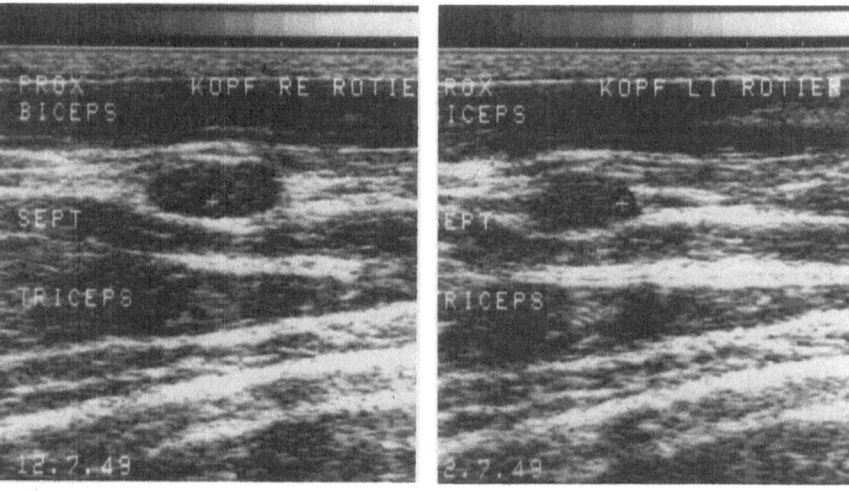

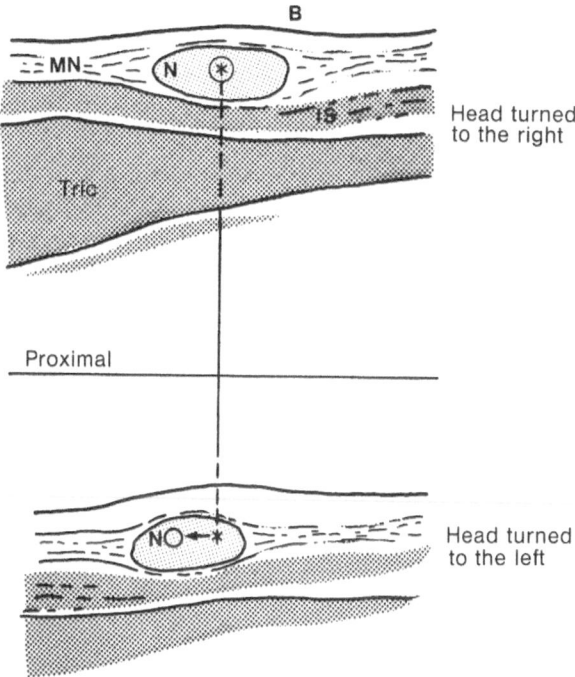

Fig. 109. Neurinoma of the right median nerve, proximal upper arm. Longitudinal AP scan of the mid-upper arm medial to the humeral shaft. The neurinoma (**N**) appears as a hypoechoic mass directly overlying the echogenic structure of the median nerve (**MN**). The triceps muscle (**Tric**) with its longitudinal striations lies below the intermuscular septum (**IS**). Above the intermuscular septum is the brachialis muscle (**B**) and the neurovascular bundle, in which the median nerve is depicted on this scan plane. Turning the head to the left *(Kopf u. Rotier)* places traction on the brachial plexus, displacing the upper portion of the median nerve proximally along with the neurinoma *(lower half of figure)*

Sonographic Anatomy

The anatomic features of individual joints were detailed in the preceding chapters. When evaluating soft-tissue structures of the musculoskeletal system in general, the examiner must become reoriented with regard to regional topographic anatomy. Easily identifiable landmarks such as blood vessels, large muscle groups, and neighboring joints are most helpful in this orientation process.

If the regional anatomy has been so altered by trauma, neoplasia, or other disease that recognition proves difficult, orientation can be aided by comparison with the unaffected contralateral side.

The different types of tissue *(fat, muscle, tendon)* have characteristic echo patterns and in some cases are separated from one another by adjacent fascia.

Blood vessels appear as hypoechoic bands that contrast well with their surroundings. Arteries are recognized by their pulsations, and many larger veins contain valves that are displayed as echogenic septa.

The fibrous septa in *fatty tissue* have no preferential orientation. Generally they appear as short linear or curvilinear echoes. Fatty tissue varies in its echo characteristics, and while most fat is only moderately echogenic, some subcutaneous fat is so echogenic that it hampers the visualization of deeper structures ("transmission loss").

Normal *muscle tissue* is hypoechoic, the bright echoes of the muscular septa indicating the direction of the muscle fibers. When the muscle is imaged longitudinally, the septa present a longitudinal and almost parallel arrangement; on transaxial scans the septa appear as points or arcs. The hyperechoic septa become more dense toward the origins and insertions of muscles and merge with the tendons.

Tendons appear hyperechoic when their axis is perpendicular to the scan plane. Tendons that are oblique in relation to the beam appear hypoechoic, an effect that increases with the degree of obliquity.

Hyaline cartilage is hypoechoic and practically devoid of internal echoes.

Bony surfaces appear as bands of high-level echoes.

Interpretive Criteria

Ultrasound can define changes in the *surface structure* of bone caused, for example, by a bony excrescence or a cortical discontinuity (e. g., an erosive defect or osteolytic lesion caused by a skeletal metastasis). With bone tumors, local elevation of the periosteum may be noted at the junction of normal and affected bone, with associated subperiosteal calcification (Fig. 110). These changes correspond to "Codman's triangles" on roentgenograms.

Soft-tissue structures are evaluated for *changes in echogenicity, discontinuities,* and *changes in shape.* Lesions that are interposed between normal structures are evaluated in terms of their extent, their delineation with respect to adjacent structures, and their echogenicity.

Degenerative changes in tendons or muscles may be associated with a change of echogenicity. It should be recalled that changes in the fiber direction of tendons or muscles produce a change of echogenicity, so these areas should always be scanned on two planes to avoid misinterpretation (see p. 9).

A change in the echogenicity of a structure has effects on underlying tissues. Thus, acoustic enhancement occurs deep to an echo-free zone while attenuation or total shadowing is observed deep to areas of increased echogenicity (see Fig. 116). Discontinuities in the substance of a tendon or muscle interrupt the bright internal echoes in the affected region, an effect seen most clearly on longitudinal scans.

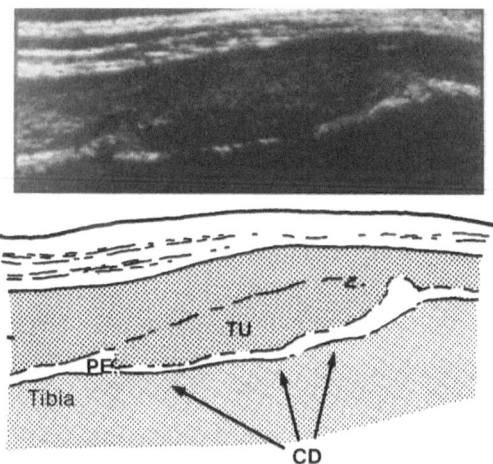

Fig. 110. Osteosarcoma of the right lower leg, longitudinal scan of the distal tibia from the anterolateral side. The extraosseous part of the osteosarcoma appears hypoechoic (**TU**). The tibia in this area shows multiple cortical discontinuities (**CD**). Periosteal elevation (**PE**) with subperiosteal calcifications is seen at the periphery of the extraosseous tumor component

Pathologic Conditions

Soft-Tissue Changes Not Caused by Trauma

Pathologic deposits in *fatty tissue* most commonly consist of gouty tophi and, in patients with rheumatoid arthritis, rheumatic nodules. The former are hyperechoic with a distal acoustic shadow, while the latter are generally hypoechoic to echo-free (see p.61).

Normal *muscle tissue* is hypoechoic with internal echoes representing muscular septa. Variations in the echogenicity of muscle do not necessarily signify disease. The muscle tissue of young, muscular patients tends to be significantly less echogenic than the muscle of older, sedentary individuals. However, intraindividual differences in muscle echogenicity can have pathologic significance (Fig. 111), as Rott showed in patients with muscular dystrophy.

Tendon tissue, being bradytrophic, is susceptible to degenerative changes. These changes are commonly observed sonographically in the supraspinatus tendon, appearing as echogenic areas that may be quite sonodense and cast a prominent shadow.

Tendon and tendon-sheath involvement in rheumatoid arthritis is manifested by the deposition of hypoechoic material in the peritendinous region (Fig. 112).

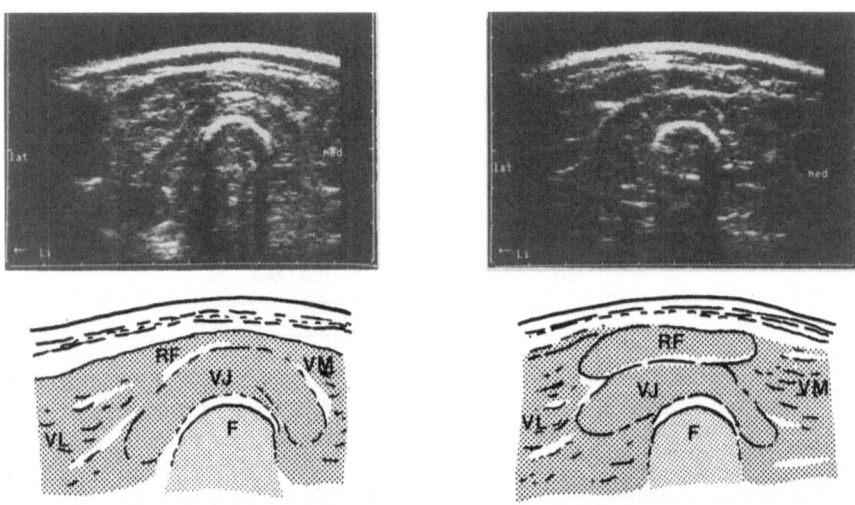

Fig. 111. Dermatomyositis. Anterior transverse scan through the center of the thigh. *Left* dermatomyositis, *right* normal thigh in a patient of equal age and similar constitution. The scan on the right clearly defines the components of the quadriceps group [rectus femoris (**RF**), vastus intermedius (**VI**), vastus lateralis (**VL**), vastus medialis (**VM**)], and the muscular septa are well delineated from the hypoechoic muscle tissue. In the left scan normal anatomic boundaries are obscured, the margins of the muscle bellies are poorly defined, and the echogenicity of the whole region is increased. **F** Femur

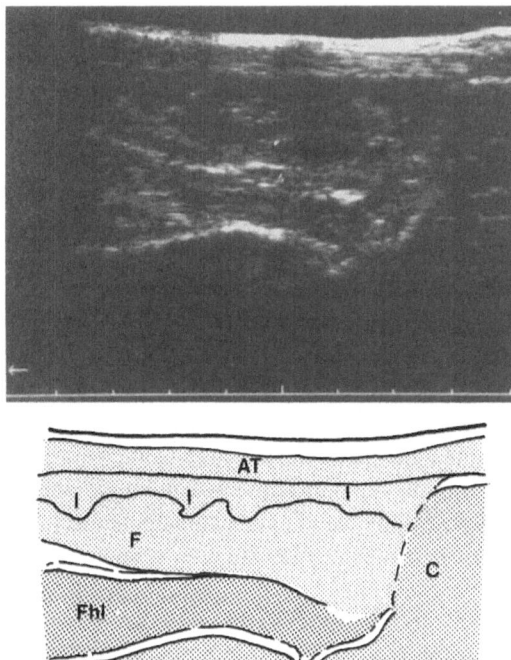

Fig. 112. Achilles peritendinitis, longitudinal scan over the Achilles tendon. The patient, known to have rheumatoid arthritis, presented with a 3-month history of swelling and redness over both Achilles tendons. Interposed between the highly echogenic tissue of the Achilles tendon (**AT**) and the less echogenic fatty tissue (**F**) is an almost echo-free zone (**I**) that is poorly demarcated from the fatty layer. It contains inflammatory proliferative tissue (**I**). **Fhl** Flexor hallucis longus, **Ti** tibia, **Ta** talus, **C** calcaneus

Posttraumatic Soft-Tissue Changes

Solid *foreign bodies* have different sound transmission properties than soft tissues, and most are easy to detect with ultrasound (Figs. 113 and 114).

The appearance of a *muscular rupture* depends on the interal elapsing between the injury and the examination.

Fresh ruptures are characterized by discontinuity of fibers and the presence of hematoma. The hematoma is hypoechoic relative to the surrounding muscle and shows distal acoustic enhancement (Fig. 115).

In older ruptures, hyperechoic scar tissue forms at the site of the tear. The echogenicity of this area is increased relative to its surroundings, and echoes from deeper structures are attenuated (Fig. 116). Calcifications forming in the scar area cast acoustic shadows (Fig. 117). This is especially marked in injuries with extensive muscle contusions and moysitis ossificans.

Fresh *tendon ruptures* are likewise characterized by a discontinuity of fiber architecture. Hematoma may expand the peritendineum and create a sharp impedance jump between the peritendineum and the tendon (Figs. 118 and 119). In dynamic scanning the ruptured ends are seen to separate as the joint bridged by the tendon is moved.

As the rupture heals, the peritendineum reapposes to the tendon tissue, and the retracted tendon stumps may be united by scar (see Fig. 37).

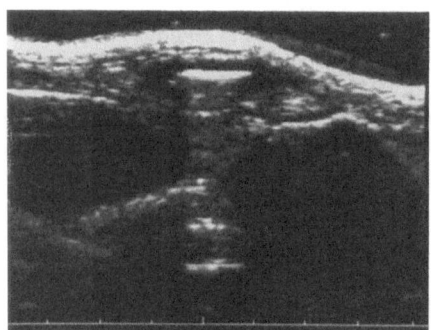 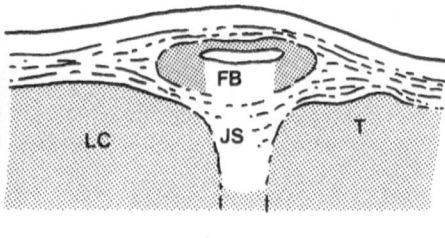

Fig. 113. Foreign body in the right knee following a motorbike accident. Sagittal scan lateral to the patellar tendon. The hyperechoic foreign body (**FB**) is lodged in the subcutaneous tissue and is surrounded by a zone of low echogenicity. It obscures the underlying joint space of the knee (**JS**). **LC** Lateral femoral condyle, **T** tibia

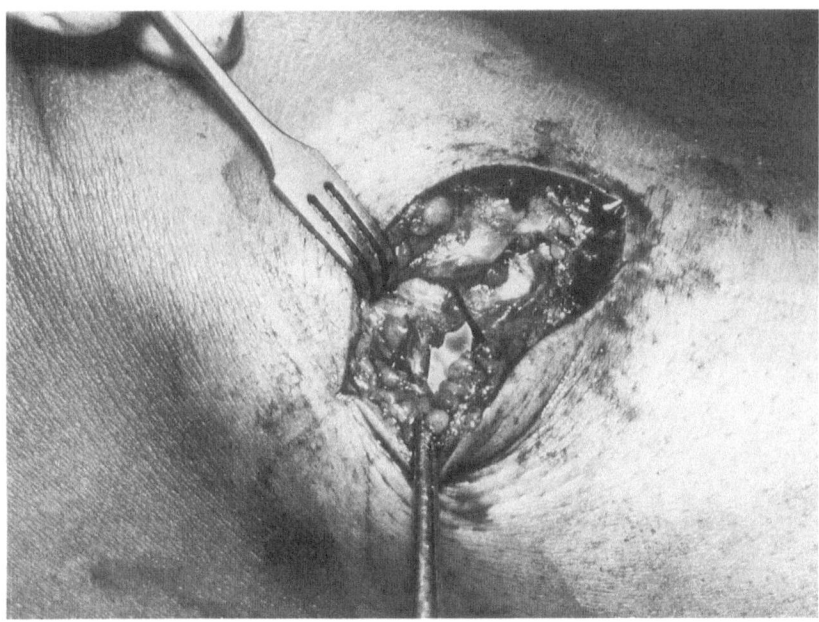

Fig. 114. Same patient as in Fig. 113, intraoperative photo showing the foreign body, a glass fragment, lying distal and slightly lateral to the patella (proximal = left)

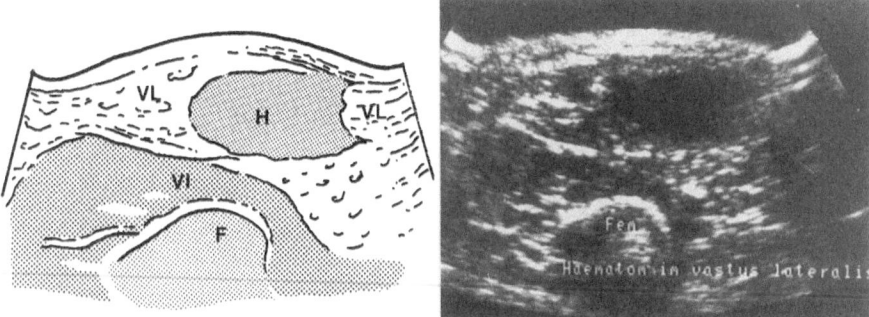

Fig. 115. Fresh rupture of the vastus lateralis. Transverse scan of the right thigh from the anterolateral aspect. The structure of the vastus lateralis (**VL**) is interrupted by a large, hypoechoic hematoma (**H**). The septa in the muscle appear as short linear echoes. **VI** Vastus intermedius, **F** femur

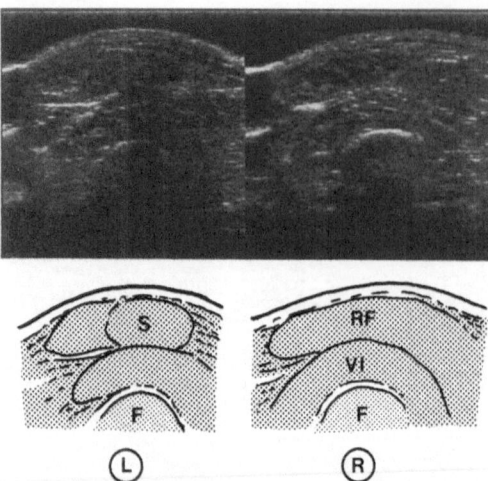

Fig. 116. Old rupture of the left rectus femoris. Transverse scan of the midthigh from the anterior side. The rupture was sustained 6 weeks earlier; the uninjured right side is shown for comparison. The scan on the left shows a homogeneous, echogenic scar (**S**) in the rectus femoris muscle (**RF**). The scar casts a faint shadow on the underlying vastus intermedius (**VI**) and femoral cortex (**F**). The echogenicity of the femur outside the scar shadow approximates that of the femur on the uninvolved side

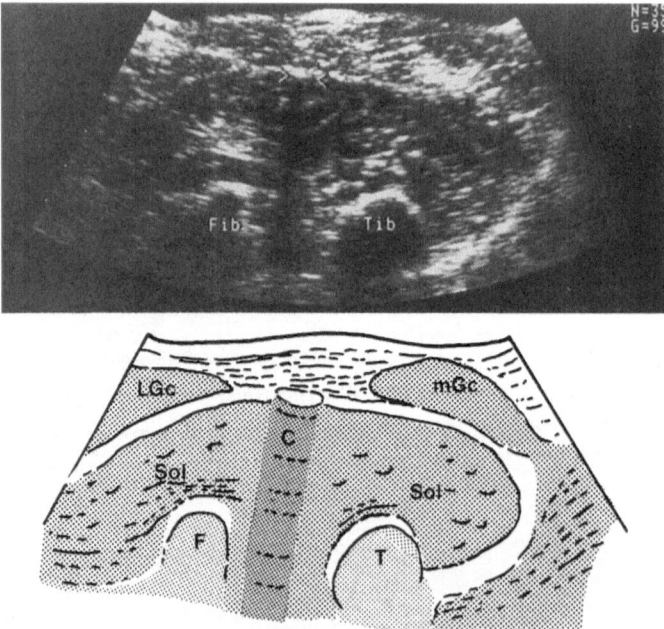

Fig. 117. Old rupture of the soleus muscle. Posterior transverse scan at the level of the calf. The soleus injury was sustained more than 2 years earlier. There is a calcification (**C**) on the superficial fascia of the soleus muscle (**Sol**) with marked distal shadowing. **LGc** Lateral gastrocnemius, **mGc** medial gastrocnemius, **F** fibula, **T** tibia

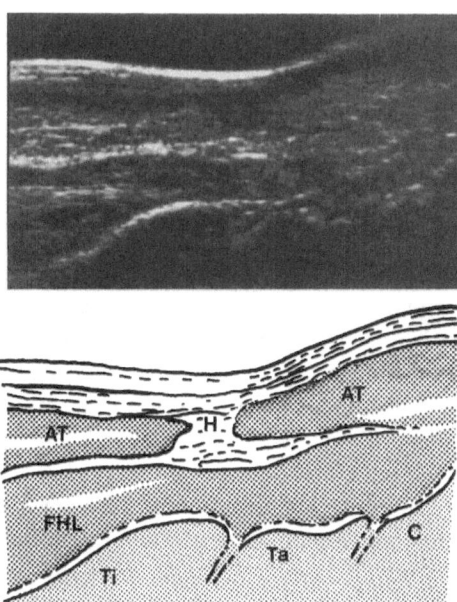

Fig. 118. Rupture of the left Achilles tendon. AP sagittal scan. The peritendineum is expanded by a hematoma (**H**), which separates the echogenic ends of the ruptured tendon (**AT**). The separation of the tendon ends is increased by flexion and extension of the ankle joint. **FHL** Flexor hallucis longus, **Ti** tibia, **Ta** talus, **C** calcaneus

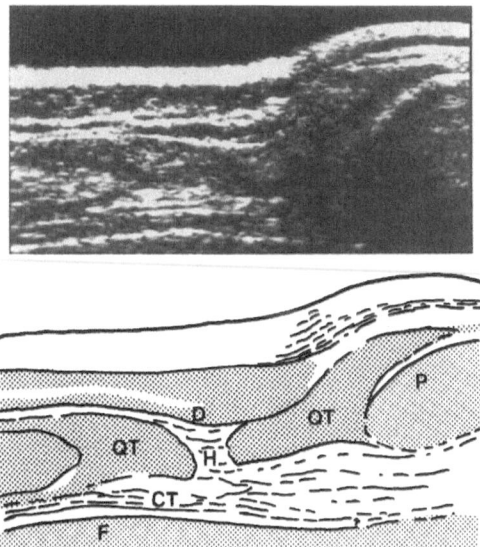

Fig. 119. Fresh rupture of the quadriceps tendon. Suprapatellar sagittal scan over the quadriceps tendon. The echogenic structure of the quadriceps tendon (**QT**) is interrupted by a hematoma (**H**). A depression (**D**) in the outer layer of the peritendineum marks the rupture site. **F** Femur, **CT** mobile connective tissue layer and synovium of suprapatellar recess, **P** patella

Space-Occupying Lesions

Most mass lesions in soft-tissue structures are readily identified owing to their *contrasting echogenicity* with surrounding tissues as well as their size and shape. This is the case with popliteal cysts, for example, which are easily recognized by their low echogenicity and the presence of a capsule (see p.99).

The cartilage portion of cartilaginous exostoses (Figs.120 and 121) is likewise hypoechoic and easily distinguished from surrounding tissues. Subcutaneous lipomas, on the other hand, have an echogenicity which closely approximates that of subcutaneous fat (Fig.122), so differentiation can be difficult. Detection is aided by demonstrating the capsule surrounding the mass.

With infiltrating tumors such as metastases from primary malignancies, delineation may be possible in areas where the tumor is separated from its surroundings by a pseudocapsule but is not possible where the tumor has invaded adjacent soft tissues without a well-defined boundary (Figs.123 and 124).

In difficult circumstances the identification of different tissue structures can be aided by performing movements during real-time scanning (see Fig.109). This is a major advantage of sonography over other imaging modalities and should definitely be utilized where necessary to aid diagnosis.

The *location* of blood vessels, especially that of arterial vessels in relation to a tumor, can generally be determined with great accuracy. Scans on multiple planes provide a good spatial impression of the size of the tumor and its relation to vascular structures (Figs.125 and 126).

Bony surfaces are evaluated to confirm or exclude the presence of cortical defects. With bone tumors, subperiosteal ossification may be noted at the junction of affected and unaffected bone (see Fig.110). These sonographic changes resemble those associated with the resumption of ossification in recovering dysplastic hips.

In the evaluation of tumors, it is important to bear in mind that the histologic type of a lesion cannot be determined from its echogenicity.

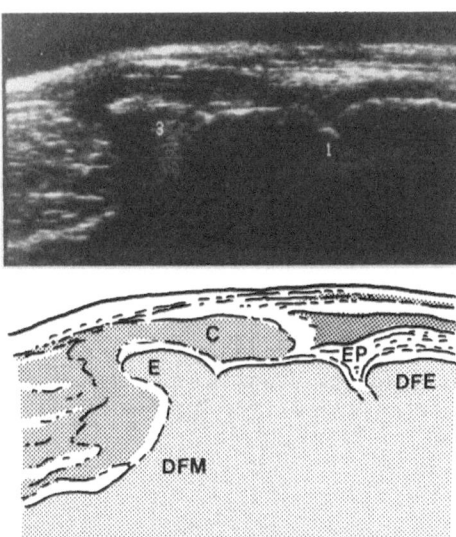

Fig. 120. Cartilaginous exostosis. Coronal scan of the right knee from the medial side. The bony part of the exostosis (**E**) casts a shadow on the distal femoral metaphysis (**DFM**), obscuring its contours. The hypoechoic cartilaginous portion of the exostosis (**C**) forms a hoodlike mass on the bony portion. **EP** Epiphyseal plate, **DFE** distal femoral epiphysis

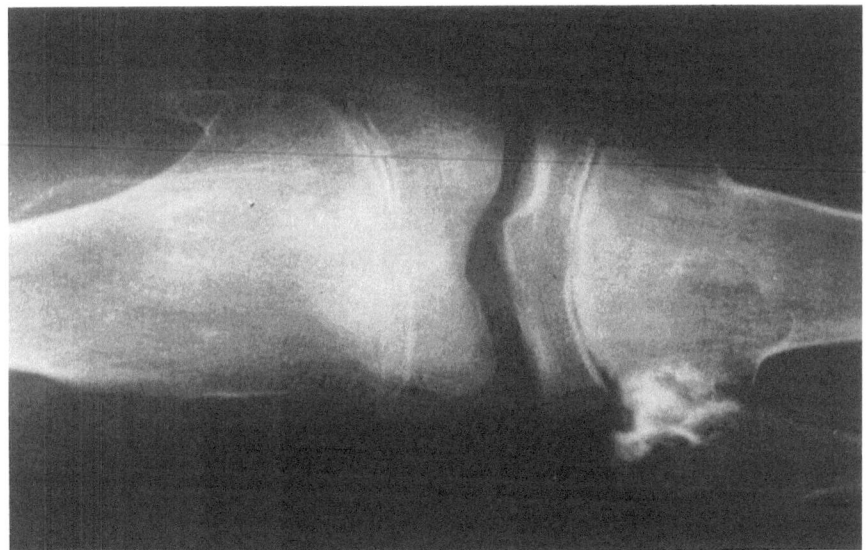

Fig. 121. Roentgenogram of the patient in Fig. 120

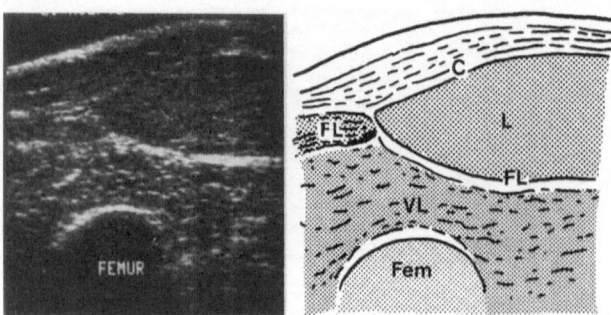

Fig. 122. Subcutaneous lipoma of the lateral thigh. Transverse scan of the proximal lateral thight. The lipoma (**L**) is isoechoic to subcutaneous fat and is surrounded by an echogenic capsule (**C**). It directly overlies the fascia lata (**FL**). The left side of the scan is anterior. **VL** Vastus lateralis, **Fem** femur

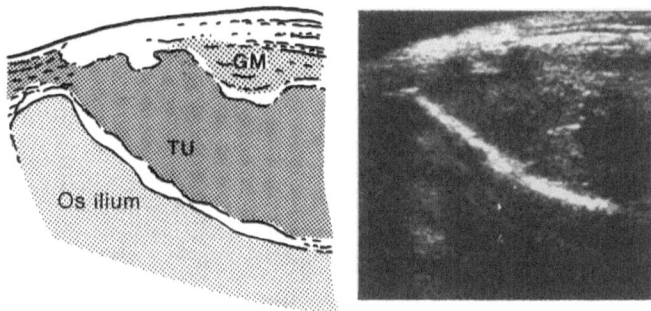

Fig. 123. Chondrosarcoma of the left ilium. Coronal scan of the left ilium from the lateral side. The tumor (**TU**) is hypoechoic with scattered higher-level echoes. It abuts directly on the surface of the ilium. The tumor is poorly demarcated from surrounding connective tissue. **GM** Gluteal muscle

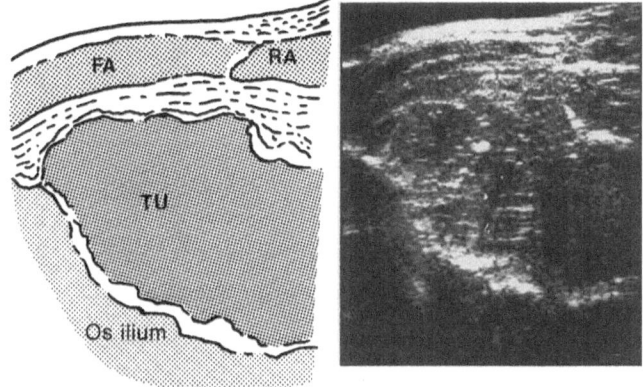

Fig. 124. Same patient as in Fig. 123. Transverse scan over the left ilium from the anterior side. The tumor (**TU**) abuts directly on the lateral surface of the ilium (see Fig. 123) and projects medially into the lesser pelvis. The mass is hypoechoic with scattered higher-level echoes. Multiple discontinuities are seen in the affected iliac cortex. The medial boundary of the tumor is also poorly defined. **FA** Flat abdominal muscles, **RA** rectus abdominis

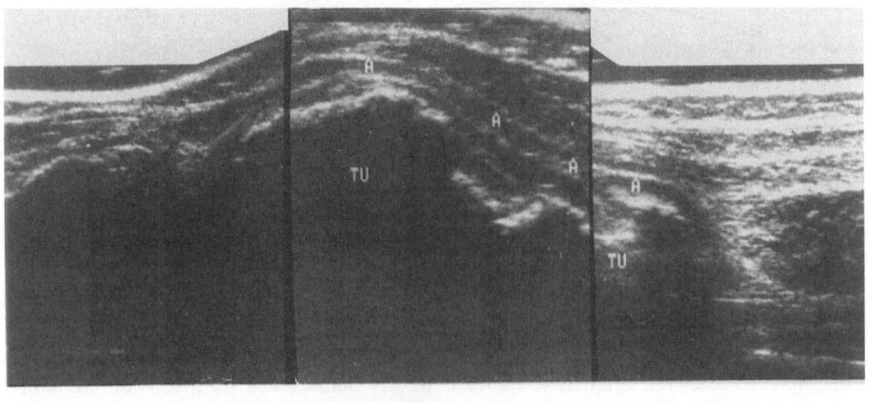

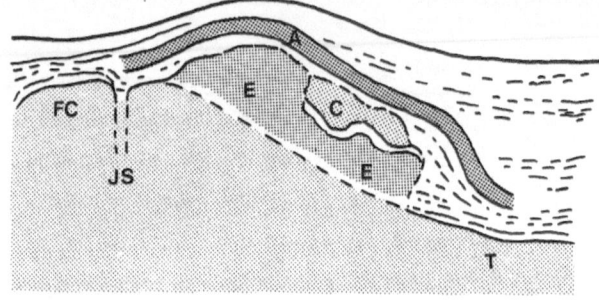

Fig. 125. Osteochondroma of the proximal tibia. Sagittal scan of the proximal tibia from the posterior side. A bulge is seen in the posterior contour of the tibia (**T**) just distal to the knee joint space (**JS**). The cartilaginous portion (**C**) of the osteochondroma is quite small compared with the osseous portion (**E**). Note the displacement of the artery (**A**) by the mass. **FC** Femoral condyle. *TU*: Tumor

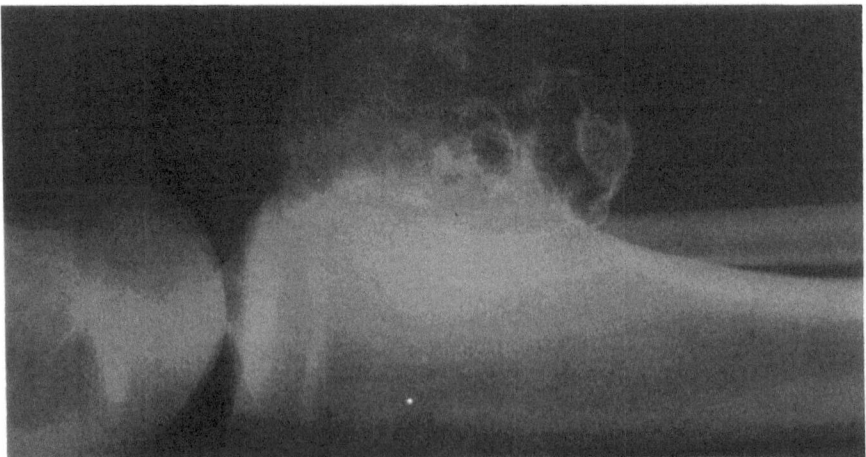

Fig. 126. Roentgenogram of the patient in Fig. 125

References

Barriga P, Garcia C (1984) Ultrasonography in detection of intra-abdominal retained surgical sponges. Z Ultrasound Med 4: 173-176

Bernadino ME et al. (1981) The extremity soft-tissue lesion: a comparative study of ultrasound, computed tomography and xeroradiography. Radiology 139: 53-59

Chivers RC, Hill RC (1975) Ultrasonic attenuation in human tissues. Ultrasound Med Biol 2: 25-29

Esche R (1952) Untersuchungen zur Ultraschallabsorption in tierischen Geweben und Kunststoffen. Akust Beiheft 2: 71-74

Fornage B (1982) Accidents musculaires du sportif. Nouv Presse Med 8: 11

Fornage BD et al. (1984) Sonography of the patellar tendon preliminary observations. AJR 143: 179-182

Frucht AH (1953) Die Schallgeschwindigkeit in menschlichen und tierischen Geweben. Z Ges Exp Med 120: 526-557

Gramberg H (1956) Absorptionsmessungen an biologischen Substanzen bei niedrigen Ultraschallfrequenzen. Dissertation, Joh.-Wolfg.-Goethe-Universität Frankfurt/M.

Kramps H-A, Lenschow E (1979) Einsatzmöglichkeiten der Ultraschalldiagnostik am Bewegungsapparat. Z Orthop 118: 355-364

Kratochwil A, Zweymüller K (1975) Ultrasound examination in orthopedic surgery. Proc 2nd Eur Congr Ultrasonics in Medicine. Experta Medica, Amsterdam, p 343

Pohlmann R (1939) Über die Absorption des Ultraschalls in menschlichen Gewebe und ihr Abhängigkeit von der Frequenz. Phys Z 40: 159-161

Seltzer SE, Finbery HJ, Weissmann BN (1980) Arthrosonography-technique, sonographic anatomy and pathology. Invest Radiol 15: 19-28

Zweymüller K, Kratochwil A (1975) Ultraschalldiagnostik bei Knochen- und Weichteiltumoren. Wien Klin Wochenschr 87: 397-398

Infant-Hip

Technique of Examination

The infant is placed on its side with the hip to be examined uppermost and flexed in a natural position. The transducer is applied at the level of the greater trochanter and oriented so that the scanning plane is approximately coronal. The "squatting" position assumed by newborns tends to redirect the pelvis and remove it from a strictly coronal plane.

Angling movements of the transducer are first used to locate the rounded, hypoechoic structure of the femoral head. Then the transducer is rotated about a transverse axis through the center of the hip joint to inspect the anterior and posterior regions of the joint. The anatomy of the hip joint is such that the femoral head has substantial bony coverage posteriorly while the anterior portions of the acetabulum are relatively flat. A correctly positioned scan will demonstrate the inferior margin of the ilium, the acetabular labrum, the superior bony rim of the acetabulum, and the site where the periosteal mantle diverges from the iliac wall. Real-time examination of the hip can provide an excellent spatial impression of the joint and how its components interrelate during movement – especially the behavior of the cartilaginous rim of the acetabulum during rotation of the femoral head and with application of tension and compression. The "standard plane" defined by Graf has indeed become the standard for image documentation. Use of this plane allows for reproducible scans and uniformity of interpretation.

Anterior or posterior deviation of the scan plane is appreciated by noting the lateral bony contour of the ilium, which should be straight and vertical. If the scan plane is too anterior, the iliac wall appears to slope outward; if too posterior, the ilium appears concave, and the bulge of the bony acetabulum can simulate good head coverage.

Normal Sonographic Anatomy (Fig. 127)

The femoral head, greater trochanter, superior cartilaginous rim of the acetabulum, and triradiate cartilage are all composed of hyaline cartilage, which appears almost echo-free because of its low acoustic impedance. Fibrous structures such as the joint capsule, periosteum, perichondrium, and acetabular labrum are more echogenic and appear as well-defined structures. The ilium, superior bony rim of the acetabulum, acetabular roof, and chondro-osseous boundary in the femoral neck and shaft form totally reflective interfaces that are intensely echogenic and shield underlying structures from view.

The highly echogenic structures of the hip help to outline the boundaries of the poorly echogenic cartilaginous structures. Thus, the superior cartilaginous rim of the acetabulum is bounded laterally by the acetabular labrum, superolaterally by the perichondrium, and medially by the ilium. Its boundary with the femoral head is occasionally defined by an intervening fluid film but is generally made clear by the geometric relationship of both structures (rounded femoral head surmounted by a triangular cartilaginous rim).

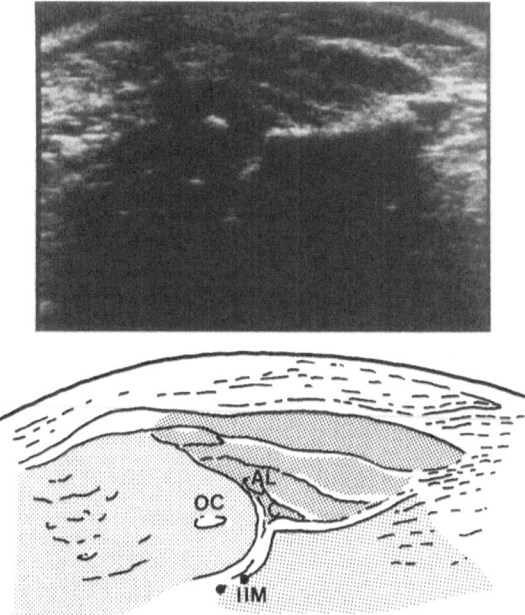

Fig. 127. Normal hip in a 5-month-old girl (Graf type I). The echo-free femoral head is composed of hyaline cartilage with a hyperechoic ossific nucleus at its center. The bony acetabulum has a sharp lateral border at its junction with the iliac wall. The inferior margin of the ilium (**IIM**) yields a bright echo and is bounded distally by the triradiate cartilage. It is bounded laterally by the superior cartilaginous rim of the acetabulum (**C**) and by the acetabular labrum (**AL**), which apposes to the medial surface of the capsule. Distal to the labrum the septa of the gluteal muscles attach to the greater trochanter. **OC** Ossification center of femoral head

Three structures should appear on the *standard imaging plane* as they are essential for evaluation of the sonogram:

- the acetabular labrum,
- the superior bony rim of the acetabulum, and
- the inferior iliac margin.

The three bones that comprise the acetabulum unite at the triradiate cartilage, which persists until puberty. The triradiate cartilage can be seen on sonograms if the ossification center of the femoral head is small and does not obscure the cartilage by its shadow. Generally this occurs after 1 year of age.

The evaluation of hip sonograms relies on defining the *inferior margin of the ilium*. On a central scan through the acetabulum, the lower iliac margin is represented by an intense echo since on this plane the bony surface is almost perpendicular to the incident beam. The ilium is bordered distally by fringes of connective tissue that stand out against the echo-free background of the triaradiate cartilage. If the scan plane is shifted anteriorly or posteriorly, the scan will enter the ascending flanges of the Y-shaped cartilage, and the iliac surface struck by the beam will become shorter and more oblique relative to the beam, causing the inferior margin to appear less sharply defined.

The *superior bony rim* of the acetabulum is the most lateral and superior part of the ossified acetabulum. Ideally this rim appears sharp and angular on the standard imaging plane. Scans anterior to the standard plane cause the rim to appear flattened, while scans posterior to the standard plane give the rim a jutting contour which gives a potentially false impression of good head containment. The superior bony rim of the acetabulum may be defined geometrically as the point of transition from the concavity of the acetabulum to the convexity of the lateral iliac wall.

The *acetabular labrum* is an echogenic structure situated between the femoral head and the joint capsule or perichondrium. It marks the lateral boundary of the cartilaginous rim of the acetabulum. It should not be mistaken for another echogenic structure which lies farther distally and laterally and represents the site of attachment of the hip capsule to the femoral neck.

Morphometry (Figs. 128-134)

Graf introduced angle measurements as a quantitative means of describing and evaluating pathologic changes in the hip joint. The α *angle* formed by the baseline and bony roof line provides a measure of the bony coverage of the femoral head. An α angle of 60° signifies good bony containment, while a smaller α angle signifies poorer coverage.

The β *angle* formed by the baseline and the cartilage roof line measures the cartilaginous coverage of the femoral head. When bony coverage is poor, a small β angle signifies compensation by the cartilaginous acetabulum. A large β angle in a hip with poor bony coverage indicates lateral migration (decentering) of the femoral head with deformation of the cartilaginous rim.

The lines that define α and β are drawn between the key anatomic structures previously described (inverior iliac margin, superior bony rim, lateral iliac wall, acetabular labrum).

The *baseline* follows the lateral wall of the ilium. It runs proximally through the point where the periosteum diverges from the bone and is tangent distally to the lateral border of the bony ilium. The *bony roof line* connects the inferior margin of the ilium with the transition point from the concavity of the acetabulum to the convexity. The *cartilage roof line* connects the transition point to the labrum.

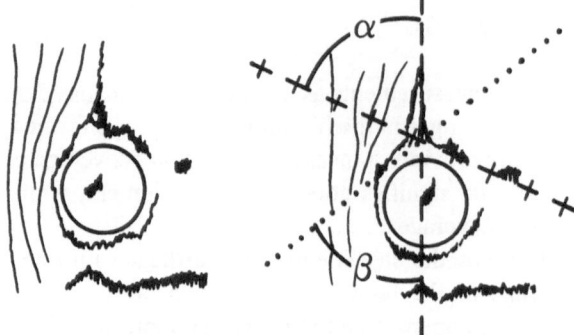

Fig. 128. Schematic illustration of the *type I hip*. The bony roof contour of the acetabulum is good, and the superior bony rim is angular. The cartilaginous rim has a narrow base and projects far over the femoral head. α is greater than 60°; β is less than 55° in type Ia and greater than 55° in type Ib. – – – – Baseline, + + + + bony roof line, ... cartilage roof line

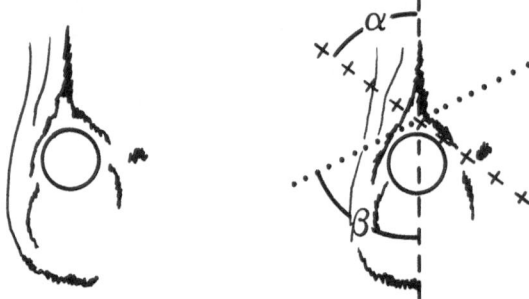

Fig. 129. Schematic illustration of the *type II hip* (a/b). The superior bony rim of the acetabulum is rounded. The cartilagenous rim surmounts the ilium on a broad base but still projects well distally over the femoral head. The head is well centered within the bony acetabulum and its cartilaginous rim. α is between 50° and 59°, β is greater than 55°. Type II represents a "physiologic delay of ossification" before 3 months of age (IIa). It is considered pathologic thereafter (IIb)

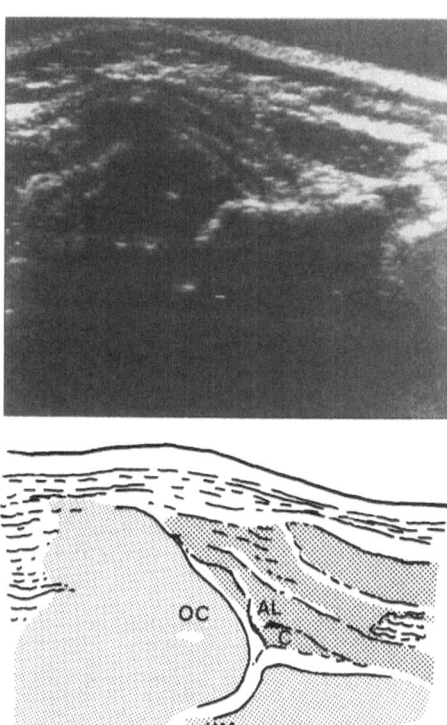

Fig. 130. Left hip of a 5-month-old girl with bilateral hip dysplasia. Left hip is type IIb. The superior bony rim of the acetabulum is rounded. The cartilaginous rim (**C**) surmounts the ilium on a broad base and is bounded laterally by the large acetabular labrum (**AL**). The femoral head is still well centered within the bony and cartilaginous acetabulum. **OC** Ossification center of femoral head, **IIM** inferior iliac margin

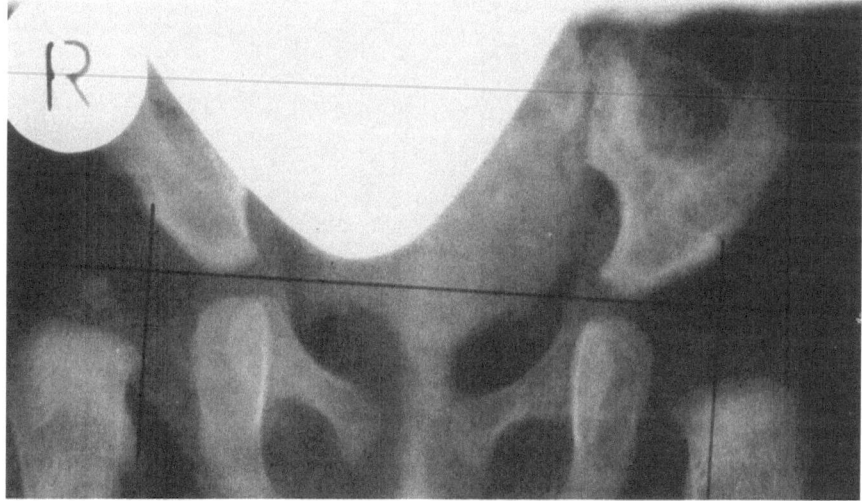

Fig. 131. Roentgenogram of the hip in Fig. 130

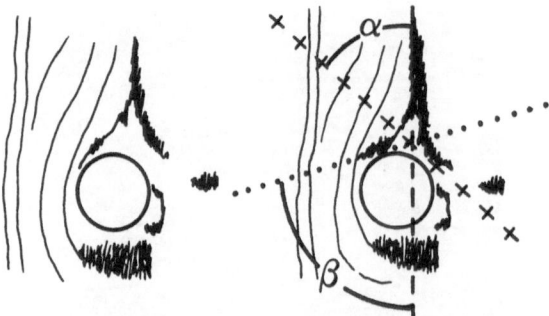

Fig. 132. Schematic illustration of the type II (c/d) hip. The superior bony rim of the acetabulum is rounded or flattened, and the cartilaginous rim surmounts the ilium on a broad base. Because of the deficient bony roof contour, compressive forces are transmitted from the femoral head to the soft cartilaginous rim, which may be displaced upward. α is between 43° and 49°, β is between 70° and 77° (type IIc). Greater compressive forces on the acetabular cartilage cause β to exceed 77° (type IId). – – – – Baseline, + + + + bony roof line, ... cartilage roof line

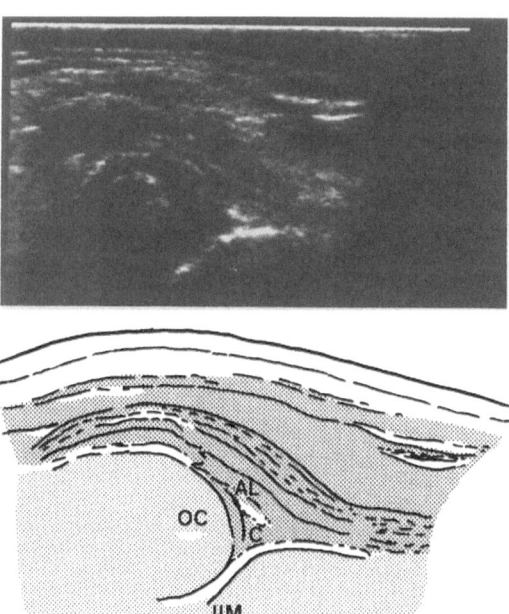

Fig. 133. Left hip of an 8-month-old girl with bilateral hip dysplasia, type IId. The bony roof contour of the acetabulum is markedly deficient, and the superior bony rim is round. The cartilagenous rim (**C**) is displaced and has approximately the shape of an equilateral triangle. The acetabular labrum (**AL**) is deflected upward by the femoral head. The capital femoral ossification center (**OC**) is struck tangentially by the beam. **IIM** Inferior iliac margin

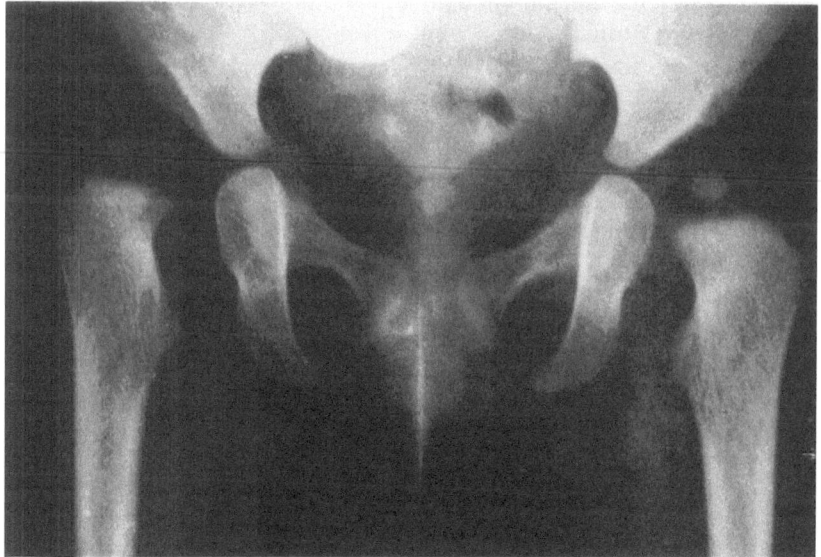

Fig. 134. Roentgenogram of the hip in Fig. 133

Classification of Sonographic Hip Findings

The α and β angles can be used to classify hips into several categories.

The *type I hip* is normal (see Figs. 127 and 128). The bony acetabulum is well defined and has an angular superior rim. The cartilaginous rim has a small base apposing to the ilium and projects well distally over the femoral head, tapering to a point. α is 60° or more, β is 55° or less. In some cases the cartilaginous rim is shorter and does not extend as far distally, so that β is greater than 55°, but this has no pathologic significance (Table 4).

Table 4. Type I hip

Subtype	α angle	β angle
Ia	$\geq 60°$	$\leq 55°$
Ib	$\geq 60°$	$> 55°$

In the *type II hip* α is between 43° and 59° and β is greater than 55°. This group is further subdivided into II a/b and II c/d according to age and degree of dysplasia.

Before 3 months of age it is common to find a slightly rounded superior bony rim accompanied by good cartilaginous coverage of the femoral head. α is between 50° and 59°, β is greater than 55°. This hip would be classified as type II a before 3 months of age (physiologic delay of ossification) and type II b after 3 months of age (see Figs. 129-131).

With increased flattening of the bony rim and upward deflection of the cartilaginous rim, α is further reduced while β is increased. Graf applied the category II c to hips with an α angle of 43°-49° and a β angle of 70°-77° and II d to hips with a β angle greater than 77° (Table 5, see Figs. 132-134).

Table 5. Type II hip

Subtype	α angle	β angle	Relation to age
IIa	50°-59°	$> 55°$	≤ 3 months
IIb			> 3 months
IIg	43°-49°	70°-77°	Independent of age
IId	43°-49°	$> 77°$	

A *type III hip* (Figs. 135-137) is characterized by further flattening of the bony acetabulum with greater widening and eversion of the cartilaginous rim. α is less than 43°, β is greater than 77°.

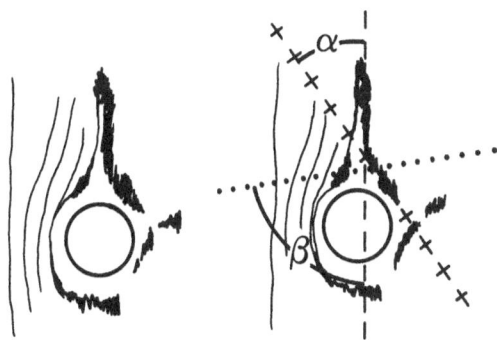

Fig. 135. Schematic illustration of *type III hip*. The bony roof contour of the acetabulum is poor, and the superior bony rim is very flat. The cartilagenous rim surmounts the ilium on a broad base and is displaced upward. α is less than 43°, β is greater than 77°. The type III hip with a normal cartilaginous rim is classified as IIIa. In the IIIb hip the cartilaginous rim has become echogenic as a result of structural change. − − − − Baseline, + + + + bony roof line, ... cartilage roof line

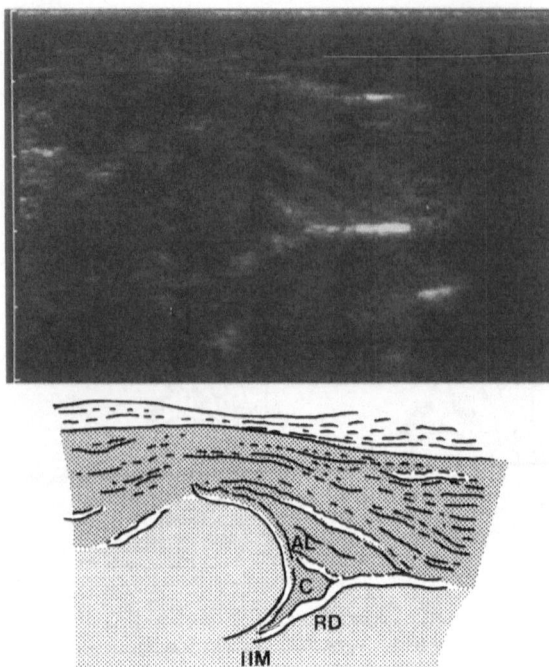

Fig. 136. Type IIIa left hip in a 3-month-old girl. The bony roof contour of the acetabulum is poor, and there is a defect in the superior bony rim (**RD**). The cartilaginous rim (**C**) surmounts the ilium on a broad base and is everted but shows no structural change. The acetabular labrum (**AL**) is deflected upward. **IIM** Inferior iliac margin

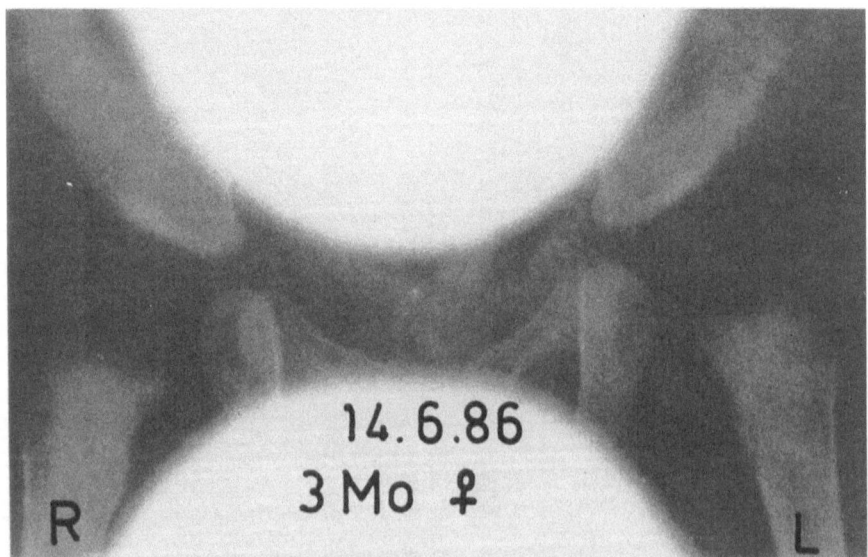

Fig. 137. Roentgenogram of the hip in Fig. 136

Distortion of the cartilaginous rim in the type III hip may progress to a point where the hyaline cartilage undergoes structural change resulting in increased echogenicity. The type IIIa hip has a normally hypoechoic, histologically unchanged cartilaginous rim, whereas the rim cartilage in the IIIb hip becomes structurally disordered and fills in with echoes (Table 6, Fig. 138). The *type IV hip* is completely dislocated (Figs. 139 and 140).

Table 6. Type III hip

Subtype	α angle	β angle	Structural changes in roof cartilage
IIIa	<43°	>77°	No
IIIb			Yes

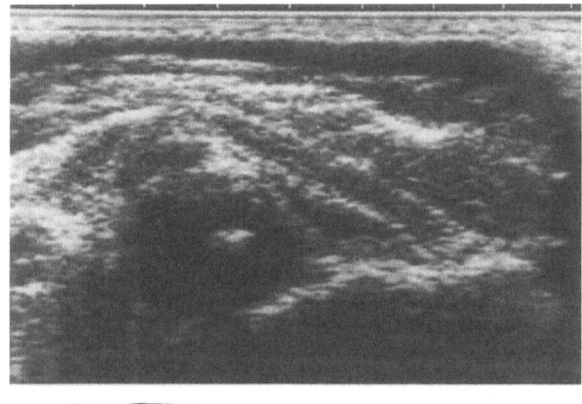

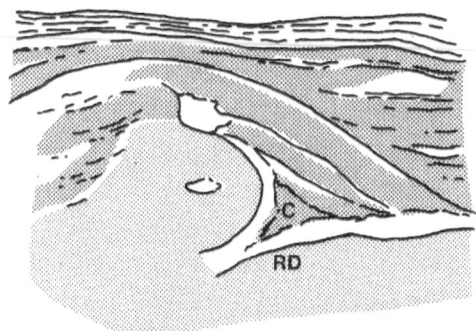

Fig. 138. Type IIIb right hip in a 5-month-old girl. The superior cartilaginous rim (**C**) is more echogenic than the underlying anechoic femoral head, and there is a defect in the lateral bony rim of the ilium (**RD**). See Fig. 131 for corresponding roentgenographic findings

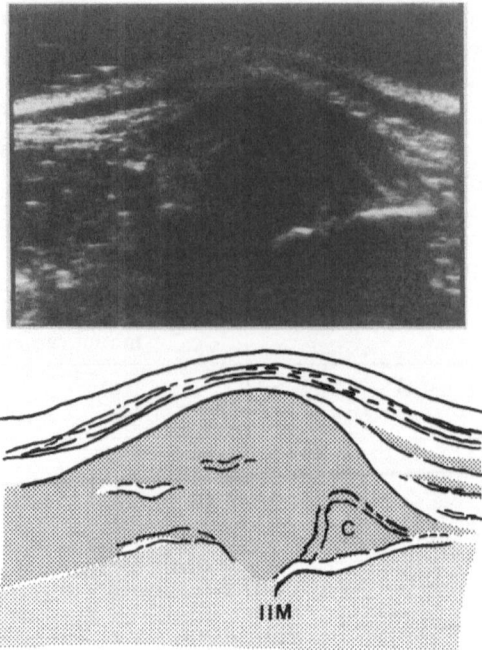

Fig. 139. Dislocated left hip in a 6-month-old girl, type IV. The bony roof contour of the acetabulum is poor, the superior bony rim is flat. The cartilaginous rim (**C**) is deformed and shows mixed hyper- and hypoechoic features. The structure of the femoral head is not visible on this scan. **IIM** Inferior iliac margin

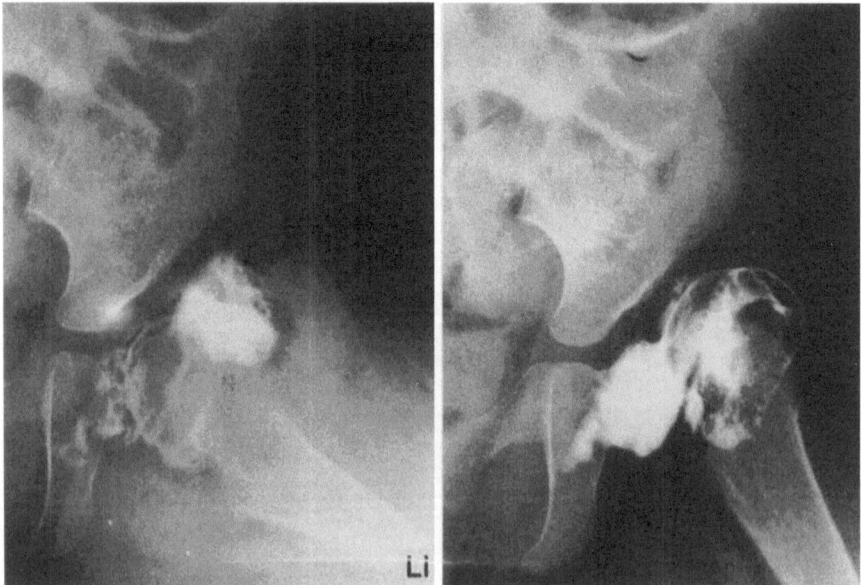

Fig. 140. Arthrogram of the hip in Fig. 139

Role of Sonography and Therapeutic Implications

Sonography is an imaging modality that is completely safe when applied within the guidelines established by the American Institute for Ultrasound in Medicine. Its indications are correspondingly broad, and it is a satisfactory method for short-term follow-ups.

An advantage of sonography over radiography in hip dysplasia is that ultrasound can demonstrate the cartilaginous anlage of structures responsible for further growth, permitting a very early diagnostic evaluation.

Hips classified as type IIc or worse usually are clinically symptomatic, and sonographic imaging serves to confirm the diagnosis. Treatment response also can be monitored with ultrasound by noting structural changes in the cartilaginous rim of the acetabulum (e.g., change from type IIIb to IIIa) and the progression of acetabular ossification.

Effective clinical follow-up is not possible in type IIa and IIb hips, and in these cases sonography offers the opportunity for very early diagnosis and a differentiated follow-up so that any deterioration can be promptly recognized.

References

Graf R (1982) Die anatomischen Strukturen der Säuglingshüfte und ihre sonographische Darstellung. Morphol Med 2: 29-38

Graf R (1983) Die Bedeutung der Sonographie bei der Untersuchung der Säuglingshüfte. Biomed Technik 28/11: 257-263

Graf R (1985) Sonographie der Säuglingshüfte. Enke, Stuttgart

Graf R, Schuler P (1986) Die Säuglingshüfte im Ultraschallbild: ein Atlas. Edition Medizin, VCH, Weinheim

Rott HD (1984) Ultraschall in der Medizin: Biologische Wirkungen und Sicherheitsaspekte. Dtsch Arztblatt 47: 1071

Joints of the Wrist

Technique of Examination

Basically two techniques are available for examination of the hands:
1. The transducer is used in conjunction with a concave standoff pad, preferably one having a variable curvature.
2. The hands are immersed in a gas-free water bath. In this technique the very high impedance jump between the water and skin produces exceptionally high-level echoes on the skin surface. (The height of the impedance jump depends on the difference in the sound transmission velocities of the adjacent media.)

The joints are actively moved during the examination to assist in the identification of specific structures. In a water bath system, the movements should be performed slowly and deliberately to minimize the echo return from turbulence.

Normal Sonographic Anatomy

Scans through the dorsal aspect of the normal hand show highly echogenic bony contours but few recognizable soft-tissue details. The skin, subcutaneous tissue, tendons, and connective tissue structures all have very similar echo characteristics in the absence of disease. While the surface contours of bony structures are well defined, the joint spaces (e. g., radiocarpal, intercarpal, carpometacarpal) can only be identified by dynamic scanning during articular movement. The distal end of the radius is relatively easy to distinguish from the scaphoid bone during movement of the radiocarpal joint. It is more difficult to separate the trapezoid and trapezium from the scaphoid on the radial longitudinal scan, because the intercarpal joint spaces are inherently more difficult to discern (Fig. 141).

Visualization of the ulnocarpal joint on the longitudinal scan shows the soft-tissue structures overlying the distal ulna, lunate, and capitate. Movements of the bones help to differentiate the individual joints. Evaluation is easier from the volar side, where the muscles improve the sound transmission.

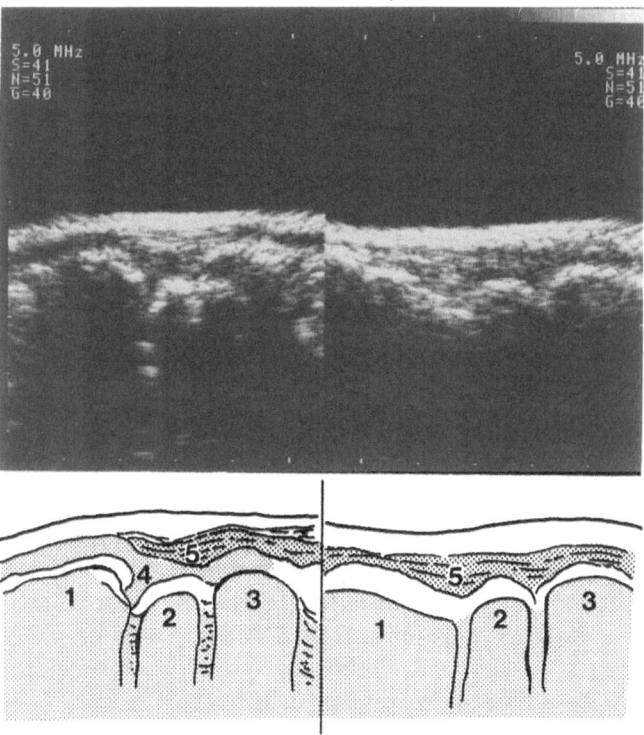

Fig. 141. Carpal arthritis in a 77-year-old man with seropositive rheumatoid arthritis, longitudinal scan over the ulna. **1** Distal end of ulna, **2** lunate bone, **3** hamate bone, **4** synovitis, **5** tendons. Normal findings are shown for comparison

Interpretive Criteria

As in other joints, inflammatory changes significantly enhance the sonographic visualization of carpal structures. While normally it is very difficult to distinguish the extensor tendeons on the dorsal side and the flexor tendons on the volar side from the surrounding retinaculum and other structures, the tendons can often be defined very clearly when tenosynovitis is present. The carpal bones also are defined more clearly when scanned through tissues involved by synovitis.

Pathologic Conditions

Carpal Arthritis

When there is inflammation of the distal or proximal carpal joints, the quality of sound transmission to the underlying bone improves with the degree of synovial thickening. Cortical echoes become more intense, and joint spaces appear sharply outlined by inflammatory substrate. Associated bone defects appear as punched-out surface discontinuities. These lesions should be imaged on two planes so they can be characterized definitively as local bone defects. It is easy to detect synovitis in the radiocarpal joint, which is best examined on longitudinal scans from the dorsal and volar sides. Inflammations of the intercarpal joints and carpometacarpal joints are also readily detected on longitudinal and transverse scans (Fig. 142).

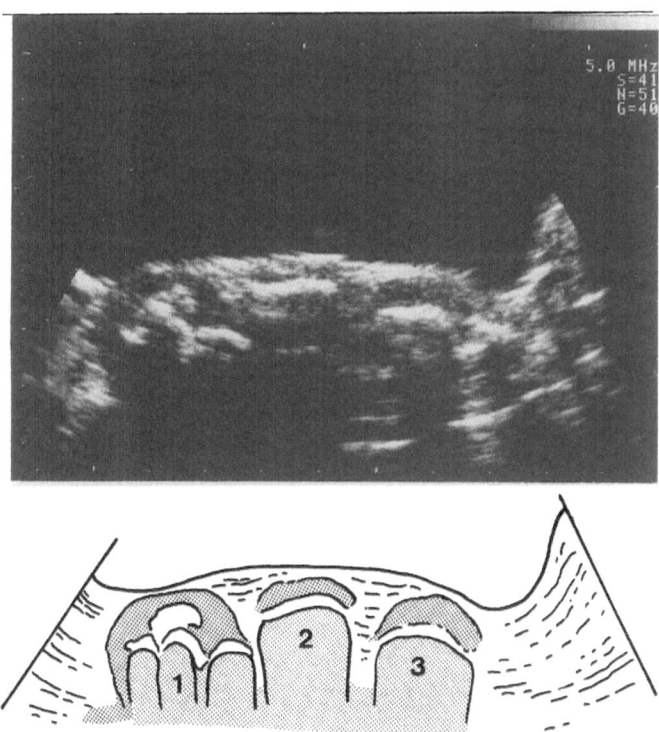

Fig. 142. Severe arthritis of the right metacarpophalangeal joints in a 77-year-old man with seropositive rheumatoid arthritis, transverse scan over the third, fourth, and fifth fingers with subluxation of the fifth finger. **1** Base of proximal phalanx of fifth finger, **2** fourth finger, **3** third finger with pronounced inflammatory substrate

Tenosynovitis

The tendon sheath thickened by inflammation appears as a tubular structure that usually can be traced for some distance along the course of the tendon. The tendon appears centrally as a very bright reflector, creating the "highway marking" appearance described previously in the ankle joint. The more extensive and severe the tenosynovitis, the greater the echogenicity of the tendon in the surrounding inflammatory substrate, in which case the tenosynovitis can usually be traced from the forearm to a point well beyond the wrist (Fig. 143).

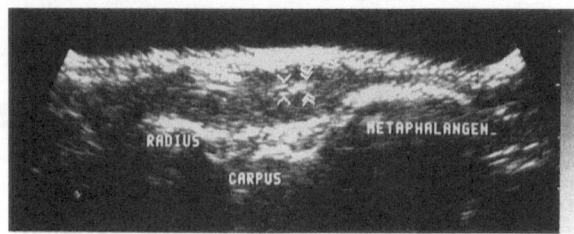

Fig. 143. Tenosynovitis of the extensor tendon over the right wrist

Ulnar Head Syndrome

Involvement of the ulnar head or styloid process in rheumatoid arthritis is frequently associated with early bone defect formation or erosive bone change that appears sonographically as a conspicuous discontinuity in the bone surface. If the styloid process or entire head of the ulna has been destroyed by multiple defects, ultrasound reveals a bizarre echo pattern that displays nothing of the original anatomy of the ulnar head. Again, the surrounding inflammatory substrate enhances sound transmission to the affected bone (Fig. 144).

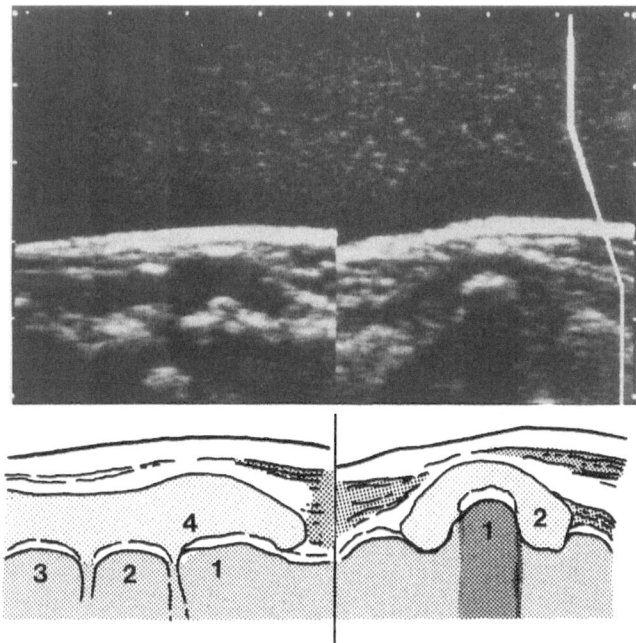

Fig. 144. *Left:* Carpal arthritis with ulnar head syndrome. Inflammatory substrate over distal and proximal carpus and over the radius, longitudinal scan over the scaphoid and trapezoid bones. 1 Radius, 2 scaphoid, 3 trapezoid, 4 inflammatory substrate. *Right:* Rheumatoid arthritis with ulnar head syndrome, transverse scan. 1 Ulnar head with acoustic shadow, 2 inflammatory substrate

Interphalangeal Joints

Synovitis of the interphalangeal joints appears on the monitor as a hypoechoic mass filling the joint space and causing enlargement of the joint. However, these changes are easily detected by palpation, and there seems to be little rationale for sonographic evaluation.

The major role of diagnostic ultrasound in the hand is in differentiating carpal arthritis from tenosynovitis and the occasional detection of destructive bone changes. It is reasonable to assume that further technical advances, including the use of higher sound frequencies, will increase and improve the information afforded by sonography and thereby justify the time expenditure of the examination.

References

Ernst J, Albrecht HJ (1984) Sonographische Darstellbarkeit des Entzündungssubstrats bei rheumatoider Arthritis. Z Rheumatol 43: 205
Ernst J (1985) Ultraschalldiagnostik in der Rheumatologie. Aktuel Rheumatol 10: 35–42
Khaleghian R, Tonkin LJ, De Geus JJ, Lee JP (1984) Ultrasonic examination of the flexor tendons of the fingers. JCU 12 (9): 547–551
Sattler H (1987) Die Arthrosonographie – Ein neues zusätzliches bildgebendes Verfahren zur Erfassung von Gelenkerkrankungen. Therapiewoche 7/87: 216

Subject Index

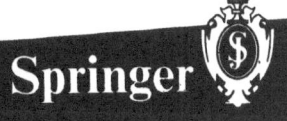

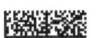